The Global HIV Epidemics among People Who Inject Drugs

The Global HIV Epidemics among People Who Inject Drugs

*Arin Dutta, Andrea Wirtz, Anderson Stanciole, Robert Oelrichs,
Iris Semini, Stefan Baral, Carel Pretorius, Caroline Haworth,
Shannon Hader, Chris Beyrer, and Farley Cleghorn*

THE WORLD BANK
Washington, D.C.

ISBN (paper): 978-0-8213-9776-3
eISBN (electronic): 978-0-8213-9777-0
DOI: 10.1596/978-0-8213-9776-3

Cover painting: "Untitled" by Raimundo Rubio, 1998. Oil on canvas, 52 by 52 in., World Bank Art Collection.

Cover design: Naylor Design

Library of Congress Cataloging-in-Publication Data
The global HIV epidemics among people who inject drugs/ by Arin Dutta ... [et al.].
 p. ; cm. -- (Directions in development)
Includes bibliographical references.
I. Dutta, Arindam, 1976- II. World Bank. III. Series: Directions in development (Washington, D.C.)
[DNLM: 1. HIV Infections--epidemiology. 2. HIV Infections--prevention & control--Statistics. 3. Substance Abuse, Intravenous--epidemiology. 4. World Health--Statistics. WC 503.41]
614.5'99392--dc23
                                                                                    2012042472

Contents

Boxes

Figures

Acknowledgments

This Economic and Sector Work was undertaken by the World Bank under the Project P124668, "The Global Epidemics of HIV among People who Inject Drugs." Support from UNAIDS under the UBW Trust Fund is gratefully acknowledged.

The project was conducted by a World Bank core team from the Health, Nutrition and Population Unit (HNP), Human Development Network: Iris Semini, Anderson Stanciole, Fazu Mansouri, and Robert Oelrichs (Task Team Leader) with the Futures Group and Johns Hopkins Bloomberg School of Public Health, Center for Public Health and Human Rights: Farley Cleghorn, Arin Dutta, Shannon Hader, Andrea Wirtz, Stefan Baral, Mike Sweat, and Chris Beyrer.

Sutayut Osornprasop and Katie Bigmore contributed to the sections on Thailand and Kenya. Additional World Bank staff members who provided technical input throughout the project include Kees Kostermans, Berk Özler, Marelize Görgens, and David Wilson. The team also thanks the following World Bank Staff for their expert and constructive criticism during the course of the work: Mai Thi Nguyen, Tekabe Belay, and Son Nam Nguyen. Thanks are also due to Nicole Klingen (Manager) and Cristian Baeza (Director) of HNP for their careful support and guidance.

We thank Jacques van der Gaag (Brookings Institution), Annette Verster, (World Health Organization), and Riku Lehtovuori (United Nations Office on Drugs and Crime) for their helpful technical inputs. Several individuals and institutions contributed data used in the case studies in this report. Gratitude is extended to Reychaad Abdool and Stéphane Ibáñez-de-Benito from the UNODC regional team in Nairobi; Dr. Faran Emmanuel and Dr. Ali Razaque from the National AIDS Control Program in Pakistan; Oussama Tawil from UNAIDS Pakistan; and Charles Vitek from CDC Ukraine, who provided input during the development of this report. We would also like to acknowledge inputs and consultation from Caroline Haworth, Rachel Sanders, Nathan Wallace, Kay Wilson, Carel Pretorius, John Stover, and colleagues at Futures Institute.

Abbreviations

AIDS	Acquired Immunodeficiency Syndrome
ANC	antenatal clinic
ART	antiretroviral therapy
ARV	antiretroviral
CDC	Centers for Disease Control
FSW	female sex worker
GHAP	Global HIV/AIDS Program
HBV	hepatitis-B virus
HCT	HIV counseling and testing
HCV	hepatitis-C virus
HIV	Human Immunodeficiency Virus
HSW	*hijra* sex worker
IBBSS	Integrated Bio-behavioral Surveillance Survey
ICER	incremental cost-effectiveness ratio
IDU	injecting drug user
LMIC	low- and middle-income countries

MAT	medically assisted therapy
MSM	men who have sex with men
MSW	male sex worker
NGO	nongovernmental organization
NSP	needle and syringe program
OST	opioid substitution therapy
PLHIV	people living with HIV
PLWHA	people living with HIV/AIDS
PWID	people who inject drugs
SGS	second generation surveillance
STI	sexually transmitted infection
UNAIDS	United Nations Joint Programme for HIV/AIDS
UNGASS	United Nations General Assembly Special Session (on HIV/AIDS)

Executive Summary

Rationale and Objectives for this Study

Recently, a set of studies published in the journal *Lancet* (July 2010 Special Issue) highlighted a neglected part of the global debate on combination prevention of HIV: interventions among people who inject drugs (PWID). This group is at higher risk for acquiring HIV infection than other adults from the general population in many countries where their populations occur. Injecting drug use is present in 148 countries (Mathers, Degenhardt et al. 2008), including a wide array of low and middle income countries (LMIC), especially some in Eastern Europe, Central Asia, and South Asia where HIV incidence is growing in recent years even as it declines elsewhere. In sub-Saharan Africa, countries such as Kenya with significant HIV epidemics in both the general and key high-risk populations now recognize the importance of PWID as a public health issue.

Despite this recognition, key harm reduction interventions that hold a strong promise of reducing risky behaviors related to transmission and acquisition of HIV are not being scaled up adequately in affected LMIC. In addition to policy barriers which limit the use of available technologies and approaches for PWID, a range of other contextual realities, including human rights abuses, abusive police practices, and widespread use of arrest, detention and incarceration, impact the health, wellbeing, and lives of PWID. A comprehensive summary of such barriers can be found in a recent publication (Strathdee, Hallett et al. 2010), as well as in Appendix B.

Improving LMIC responses requires expanding services for PWID where relevant and addressing their exclusion from key emerging interventions, such as expanded voluntary HIV counseling and testing and access to treatment. This report seeks to inform these responses by serving the following key objectives:

- Provide economic evidence for certain interventions with PWID—though cost, impact and policy analysis—that promotes a global push to reduce unmet need for services for people who inject drugs.

- Disseminate and publicize the analysis in collaboration with WHO, UNAIDS, UNODC, the International AIDS Society, and networks of PWID to maximize its impact on country policymakers.

- Create a body of knowledge and expert opinion from the analysis that can be used in continuing advocacy with stakeholders and community, e.g., explanation of the results of the study and acting as a resource to policymakers at the World Bank, donors, and governments.

This report addresses research questions related to an increase in the levels of access and utilization for four key interventions that have the potential to significantly reduce HIV infections among PWID and their sexual and injecting partners, and hence morbidity and mortality in LMIC. These interventions are drawn from nine consensus interventions that comprise a 'comprehensive package' for PWID. The four interventions are:

1. Needle and Syringe Programs (NSP)

2. Medically Assisted Therapy (MAT)

3. HIV Counseling and Testing (HCT)

4. Antiretroviral Therapy (ART)

> **Box ES.1   Why We Focus on the Four Key Interventions**
>
> This report focuses on improving HIV prevention by scaling up interventions among people who inject drugs (PWID). Based on a review of the literature (summarized in Chapter 1), four interventions had the strongest effects in this context and were picked for analysis. Stand-alone condom interventions were not included. Condom distribution does occur within the context of an effective needle and syringe program. Condoms are effective in preventing sexual transmission among PWID as well as with their sexual partners. However, this pathway of effect has been systematically reviewed and modeled elsewhere.
>
> *Source:* IOM 2007; Weller & Davis-Beaty 2007.

In this report, we summarized the results from several recent reviews of studies related to the effectiveness of the four key interventions in reducing risky behaviors in the context of transmitting or acquiring HIV infection. We look at the association between HIV outcomes (prevalence or incidence) and expanding the key interventions in isolation, especially NSP and MAT, or in combination. Overall, the four key interventions have strong effects on the risk of HIV infection among PWID via different pathways, and this determination is included in the documents proposing the comprehensive package of interventions (WHO, UNODC et al. 2009; IDU Reference Group 2010).

We use the results of this review of effectiveness in the context of HIV prevention in several case studies, and in each case study we provide an overall epidemiological overview that highlights key recent developments in the epidemic and in the country's response. For each case, we conduct a model-based analysis of the effect of scaling-up the four key interventions in combination.

Case Study Analysis

This report conducts a review of recent systematic reviews of the four key interventions initial group of countries that represented a diverse selection across PWID-HIV epidemic contexts. They represent a sub-Saharan epidemic context (Kenya), Eastern Europe and its established HIV epidemics among PWID (Ukraine), South Asia and its developing epidemics among PWID (Pakistan), and Southeast Asia with its mature HIV epidemics among PWID (Thailand).

For each case study, the modeled time period for expansion of coverage of the four key interventions was 2012–2015, and the base year was 2011. The following research questions were used for the modeling component of each case study.

a. What is the impact on HIV incidence of implementing the key interventions at a level of coverage eliminating a substantial portion of the unmet need?

b. What is the cost of expanding the key interventions to eliminate the unmet need? Based on direct effects, what is the cost-effectiveness of the expansion?

c. What is the uncertainty around costing and cost-effectiveness results for implementation of the four key interventions and how can these uncertainties best be addressed?

We use the Goals mathematical model to conduct the analysis. This model has been utilized in multiple studies over the last decade, including for a similar report on MSM. For each country case study, we model the following scenarios:

- **Status Quo:** No change in the coverage of ART, NSP, MAT, or HCT for PWID over the years 2011–15.

- **Baseline:** In this scenario the increase from levels of coverage of NSP, MAT, and HCT for PWID from the base year of 2011 across the period 2012–2015 is as per existing national plans. This coverage over 2012–2015 may be the same as the level in 2011 if we foresee no meaningful expansion or if plans do not call for increase. In this scenario, ART coverage increases every year over 2012–2015 based on the country's current scale-up plan for adult treatment. The Baseline scenario assumes that PWID have proportionate access to ART slots as the intervention scales up.

• **Expansion:** This scenario involves a scale-up of levels of provision of NSP, MAT, and HCT for PWID beyond national plans

We consider two different levels of effectiveness of NSP, MAT, and HCT for PWID in reducing risky behaviors among PWID. This form of sensitivity analysis suggests the following scenarios overall:

Status Quo	+	Conservative Impact Matrix	1. Status Quo Scenario
Baseline Scenario	+	Conservative Impact Matrix	2. Baseline Scenario
Expansion Scenario	+	Conservative Impact Matrix	3. Expansion Conservative Scenario
		Optimistic Impact Matrix	4. Expansion Optimistic Scenario

Results

Over the period from 2011–15, impressive reductions in the number of new HIV infections among PWID were observed when highly effective PWID and ART programs were expanded to ambitious yet achievable targets, in comparison to a status quo for these four interventions. Specifically, we observed in Ukraine a 34 percent reduction, Pakistan– 33 percent, Thailand– 35 percent, and Kenya– 56 percent.

We investigated a policy decision many countries face—should they consider the combination package of four interventions or just continue with ART scale-up in which PWID can gain a proportional share? In this context we again looked at the impact in terms of HIV incidence. With such combination expansion and high effectiveness, countries could avert significant number of HIV infections compared to ART alone over 2012 to 2015: Ukraine: 3,900, Pakistan: 4,130, Thailand: 1,570, and Kenya 1,300. Table ES1 summarizes the cost-effectiveness.

Table ES.1   Incremental Cost-effectiveness Ratios (ICER) of Policies Spanning 2012–15, US$ per Adult HIV Infection Averted

Case Study	Scaling Up Combination Prevention (NSP, MAT, HCT, and ART[a]) Compared to Status Quo[b]	Scaling Up Combination Prevention Compared to just Scaling Up ART[a,c]
Ukraine	$598–$5,105	$6,732–$9,221
Pakistan	$520–$8,299	$9,848–$15,300
Thailand	$404–$788	$5,403–$6,819
Kenya	$1,459–$1,600	$13,166–$19,412

Source: Authors.
Note: ART = antiretroviral therapy; HCT = HIV counseling and testing; MAT = medically assisted therapy; NSP = needle and syringe program.
a. ART scale-up with equi-proportionate access to PWID in the number of treatment slots.
b. Range based on two policies: first, scaling up ART and offering PWID an equi-proportionate share in treatment slots; second, a scale-up of all four key harm reduction interventions (including ART with equal share).
c. Range shown here is based on variation in the modeled effectiveness of individual policies, and as captured in the Goals model impact matrix.

Policy Implications and Recommendations

The results of this study demonstrate some key realities for the future of the global response to HIV. The findings presented here make clear that an 'AIDS free generation' will not be possible unless HIV prevention, treatment, and care are taken to scale for PWID. To truly begin to control the global spread of HIV, expansion, not contraction, of these services will be required. In this light, the December 2011 re-instatement of the U.S. Federal ban on funding for needle and syringe exchanges is a substantial setback for scale-up efforts in the global response.

An additional and substantive concern for efforts to address HIV among PWID has been the cancellation of Round 11 funding of the Global Fund to Fight AIDS, TB, and Malaria (GFATM). The GFATM has been a critical donor for countries with concentrated epidemics, particularly in Asia and the Former Soviet Union.

The urgency for scaling up combined prevention and treatment efforts for PWID is all the more compelling as the results of this study demonstrate that such efforts are not only effective, but cost-effective. While we did not conduct specific fiscal space analysis, we believe that the scale-up of well-targeted PWID interventions should occur within the existing context of allocations to the HIV/AIDS response in LMIC, and given the totality of priorities for prevention, treatment, and care.

Responding to HIV among PWID is highly desirable from public health and human rights perspectives. From a public health perspective, increasing investment in prevention among key high-risk groups where current investments are disproportionate to the disease burden, accords with the most basic principles of the field—high burden populations must receive efforts commensurate with disease prevalence and incidence for public health efforts to succeed. Ignoring significant populations at risk is an approach which will undermine any public health effort. From a human rights perspective the imperatives are equally compelling.

Taken together, findings indicate the need for a radically different course and set of resource allocations for HIV prevention and care among PWID. Specifically, results indicate that:

- HIV prevalence is significantly higher across four diverse geographic settings among PWID than in the general adult population; yet service coverage levels for key harm reduction interventions with HIV prevention benefits are generally low, especially for MAT. Currently, ART coverage among PWID is extremely low, which reflects the marginalized and stigmatized nature of this group.

- HIV transmission dynamics can be significantly reduced among PWID and in most cases, in extension among the general population, by well-targeted scale-up of the four key harm reductions: NSP, MAT, and HCT for PWID, as well as equi-proportionate access in ART scale-up. Countries may consider any of these interventions alone or in a subset when approaching a stepwise scale-up. For example, we specifically analyzed scaling up ART first and providing access to PWID on an equi-proportionate basis as a step in this overall scale-up path.

- In order to attain the greatest effect from these interventions, structural issues must be addressed, especially the removal of punitive policies targeting PWID in many countries.

- Research is needed that further documents the ongoing, increased social vulnerability of PWID across settings and investigates the implementation design and effectiveness of stand-alone or combination provision of key harm reduction interventions such as from the comprehensive package of nine interventions (above and beyond the four we have highlighted).

The scientific evidence presented here, the public health rationale, and the human rights imperatives are all in accord: we can and must do better for PWID. The available tools are evidence-based, right affirming, and cost effective. What is required now is political will and a global consensus that this critical component of global HIV can no longer be ignored and under-resourced.

CHAPTER 1

Background

Introduction—A Situation Update

The global epidemics of HIV among people who inject drugs (PWID) in 2012 do present challenging paradoxes for those concerned with global HIV/AIDS responses. There is abundant evidence demonstrating that the available array of prevention and treatment technologies can control parenteral transmission at individual, network, and community levels among PWID (Beyrer, Baral et al. 2010).

Yet the political, social, and legal environments in which these epidemics too often occur serve as potent barriers to program initiation, implementation, quality, and scale (Beyrer, Malinowska-Sempruch et al. 2010a; Strathdee, Hallett et al. 2010). Among opioid dependent injectors, medically assisted therapy with methadone and/or buprenorphine has been shown to reduce incident HIV infection, decrease needle and syringe use, and reduce an array of dependence related behaviors including criminal activity, unemployment, and recidivism to incarceration (Institute of Medicine 2007). However, this effective approach remains controversial in many settings, particularly in the Former Soviet Union (FSU), and in Russia, where all medically-assisted therapy other than using naltrexone remains illegal (Judice 2012).

Another paradox has been the potent and now well described impact of the provision of sterile injecting equipment to PWID, and the utility of the most common approach to this provision–needle and syringe exchange programs, or NSP (Degenhardt, Mathers et al. 2010). The data are compelling that this simple intervention can have profound impacts on HIV spread at individual and network levels—yet it was vigorously opposed by the United States for many years, with a federal ban on funding for NSP—a policy which had widespread effects on limiting the use of this intervention. In late 2011, the U.S. federal ban on funding for needle and syringe exchanges was re-imposed, returning the United States to earlier policy.

And while treatment with antiretroviral therapy (ART) has not been demonstrated to date to reduce HIV transmission from HIV-infected PWID to their injecting partners, the biological plausibility is very high that ART will act similarly for sexual transmission in this population as it has now been shown to do with high efficacy for heterosexual transmission. Yet here again, Wolfe, et al., have shown convincingly that access to ART is markedly reduced among PWID in five of the most affected countries (Russia, Ukraine, China, Malaysia, and Vietnam) limiting the potential prevention impact of this treatment modality, and increasing morbidity and mortality for PWID compared to other persons with HIV in the same countries (Wolfe, Carrieri et al. 2010).

The October, 2011 decision of the Board of the Global Fund to Fight AIDS, Tuberculosis, and Malaria (GFATM) to cancel its upcoming Round 11 funding, due to insufficient funds, further complicates the prevention and treatment access issues for PWID. Countries with concentrated epidemics in PWID in multiple regions, including those in Central, South, and Southeast Asia are heavily dependent on the GFATM. The inability to expand services due to the Global Fund limits will impose a disproportionate burden on PWID.

The limited use of available prevention and care options for PWID across affected regions have led this neglected component of global AIDS to continue to expand. In the UNAIDS Report on the Global AIDS Epidemic (2010) changes in HIV incidence between 2001 and 2009 were evaluated, and most countries were found to have epidemics either in decline or in stable states of transmission. The PWID-driven epidemics of Central Asia were a marked exception, with several states having greater than 25 percent overall increases in HIV infection (UNAIDS 2010). Overall in some 19 countries worldwide, PWID bear 20 percent or more of the overall HIV disease burden. These states include Azerbaijan, Canada, China, Estonia, Georgia, Indonesia, Italy, Kazakhstan, Kyrgyzstan, Malaysia, New Zealand, Pakistan, Russian Federation, Spain, Tajikistan, Ukraine, Uzbekistan and the United States (UNAIDS 2010).

Worldwide some 15.9 million persons (11 to 21.2 million) were estimated to be PWID in 2010 (Beyrer, Malinowska-Sempruch et al. 2010a). Figure 1 shows the global distribution of PWID and HIV prevalence.

The largest numbers of PWID are in Southeast and East Asia with approximately 4.5 million PWID, followed by Eastern Europe with an estimated 3 million PWID. In the former region, China is estimated to represent a majority of the PWID (2.3–2.9 million), followed by Japan and Indonesia. In Eastern Europe, Russia and Ukraine represent the bulk of PWID North America has over 2.2 million PWID, Latin America and Western Europe may each have over around 1 million estimated PWID. The total number of PWID across the Middle East, sub-Saharan Africa, and in South Asia is not well understood. However, it is estimated that just in Kenya (see case study in this report), Mauritius, and South Africa combined there may be about 300–350,000 PWID in Africa (Mathers, Degenhardt et al. 2008). Most PWID in Latin America, and many in North America, inject cocaine and other stimulants, rather than opiates, limiting drug treatment options for PWID in these regions. This is truly a global component of HIV, which spares no region.

Table 1.1   Estimated Numbers of PWID and Regional Prevalence of HIV among PWID, 2010

Regions	Estimated Numbers of PWID: Range[a]	Average Regional HIV Prevalence among PWID
East and Southeast Asia	4,302,943–5,030,684	15%–<20%
Eastern Europe	2,730,907–2,941,518	≥ 20%
North America	2,144,341–2,965,031	15%–<20%
Western Europe	959,124–1,028,888	5%–<10%
Latin America	908,005–909,334	≥ 20%
South and Central Asia	756,230–850,051	10%–<15%
Australasia	169,754–231,356	<5%

Source: Mathers, Degenhardt et al. 2008; Beyrer, Malinowska-Sempruch et al. 2010a.
Note: PWID = people who inject drugs.
a. Mid to upper estimates. Regional totals are based on countries with data, and hence may be an underestimate due to missing information.

A recent trend of concern is that heroin use, injection of heroin, and HIV associated with injecting, is emerging in the already high HIV burden region of East Africa (Mathers, Degenhardt et al. 2008; Baral, Trapence et al. 2009; Beyrer, Malinowska-Sempruch et al. 2010a). Outbreaks of HIV among PWID have now been reported in Kenya, Pakistan, Tanzania, Mauritius and Libya, and injecting drug use has been reported in Nigeria, Malawi, Namibia, Botswana and South Africa. African health systems, already burdened with HIV, are ill-equipped to deal with this next phase of HIV infection.

In addition to policy barriers that have limited the use of available technologies and approaches for PWID, a range of other contextual realities, including human rights abuses, abusive police practices, and widespread use of arrest, detention, and incarceration, had an impact on the health, wellbeing, and lives of PWID (Jürgens, Csete et al. 2010). Some of these barriers are summarized in Appendix B.

Box 1.1   Estimated Numbers of PWID Globally: Sources of Data

The IDU Reference Group collects and analyses global data on injecting drug use and HIV. The Reference Group's most recent substantive update of global data on numbers of PWID by country was conducted in 2008.
www.idureferencegroup.unsw.edu.au

In addition, the following sources can be consulted:

1. **Multi-country:** *Global epidemiology of injecting drug use and HIV among people who inject drugs: a systematic review* (Mathers, Degenhardt et al. 2008)

2. **South and Southeast Asia:** *A situation update on HIV epidemics among people who inject drugs and national responses in South-East Asia Region* (Sharma, Oppenheimer et al. 2009)

3. **Europe:** Ch.6 - Opioid use and drug injection in the report *'The State of the Drugs Problem in Europe'* (EMCDDA 2010)

Sources: Mathers, Degenhardt et al. 2008; Sharma, Oppenheimer et al. 2009; EMCDDA 2010.

Many of these abuses, including police brutality, have been shown to increase HIV risks by limiting PWID access to services, syringe exchanges, and drug treatment (Beyrer, Malinowska-Sempruch et al. 2010a). These approaches are costly, widespread, and generally have political support as being "tough on crime," and as components of the international "War on Drugs." But they have arguably limited the evidence-based and rights-affirming approaches of harm reduction, universal access to ARVs for people living with HIV, and access to effective drug treatment services for those PWID seeking to become drug free. Incarceration has not been shown to decrease drug use risks for PWID, but has been shown to increase sexual exposure risks for male PWID, demonstrating its failure as an HIV intervention (Degenhardt, Mathers et al. 2010).

Are there better and more cost-effective ways to address HIV among PWID? This report seeks to address the epidemiology and the cost-effectiveness of an optimal package of combined services for PWID. This includes substitution therapy for opioid-dependent PWID who want it, NSP, and expanded access to ART for PWID living with HIV. Taken together, these evidence-based and humane approaches could have a profound impact on PWID and their communities. As the global community moves to universal access and seeks to "turn the tide" on HIV with new approaches and technologies, we cannot afford to continue to ignore these populations. HIV epidemics among PWID continue to expand in 2012, and to expand to new regions. This must change, and it can be changed.

Improving low- and middle-income countries' (LMIC) responses to HIV/AIDS requires expanding services for PWID where relevant and addressing their exclusion from key emerging interventions, such as expanded voluntary counseling and testing and earlier access to HIV treatment. This report seeks to inform these responses by posing and attempting to answer several key questions. Answering the research questions serves the following key objectives:

- Provide economic evidence for certain interventions with PWID through cost, impact and policy analysis to promote a global push to reduce unmet need for services for people who inject drugs.

- Disseminate and publicize the analysis in collaboration with WHO, UNAIDS, UNODC, the International AIDS Society, and networks of people who inject drugs to maximize its impact on country policymakers.

- Create a body of knowledge from the analysis that informs expert opinion and can be used in continuing advocacy with stakeholders and community. The results of the study can act as a resource to policymakers at the World Bank and other donors, as well as in governments.

This report contains several elements that inform these policy objectives. We conduct a review of reviews of published evidence on effectiveness of certain harm reduction interventions among PWID. Using modeling, we address several research questions related to increasing the levels of provision for key highly effective harm reduction interventions that have the potential to significantly reduce HIV infections among PWID and their sexual and injecting partners, and hence morbidity and mortality in LMIC. This modeling analysis is conducted in the form of case studies. Synthesis of these modeling results, alongside policy analysis, helps us make recommendations for the overall scale-up of harm reduction interventions among PWID based on evidence.

We consider interventions from a set of nine consensus interventions identified by international stakeholders as being highly relevant in epidemics of HIV among PWID (WHO, UNODC et al. 2009; IDU Reference Group 2010). The nine interventions comprise a "comprehensive package" for PWID. Of the nine, we consider four key interventions:

1. Needle and syringe programs (NSP)

2. Medically assisted therapy (MAT)

3. HIV counseling and testing (HCT)

4. Antiretroviral therapy (ART)

These key interventions were selected because they have the strongest effects on the risk of HIV infection among PWID via different pathways. This determination is included in the documents proposing the comprehensive consensus package of interventions (WHO, UNODC et al. 2009; IDU Reference Group 2010), which summarize the results from a use of HASTE criteria—the Highest Attainable Standard of Evidence. Stand-alone condom interventions were not included. Condom distribution does occur within the context of an effective needle and syringe program. Condoms are effective in preventing sexual transmission among PWID as well as with their sexual partners. However, this pathway of effect has been systematically reviewed and modeled elsewhere (IOM 2007, Weller & Davis-Beaty 2007).

Other studies have noted that these four interventions—NSP, MAT, HCT, and ART—are highly efficacious, effective in typical scenarios of programs implemented in low and middle income countries, and have plausible outputs that can be related to reduction of risky behavior among PWID related to a risk of HIV infection. These effects of the interventions are discussed in Section 1.4.

In addition to the modeled effect on HIV incidence and related morbidity and mortality among PWID and their sexual partners, there is evidence that these interventions can reduce drug-use related morbidity and mortality, such as from overdose.

Global Coverage of the Four Key Interventions among PWID

Coverage for NSP and MAT globally has been recently surveyed by the UN Reference Group, and reported in a major review (Mathers, Degenhardt et al. 2010). Under the overall umbrella of harm reduction interventions, a global review of coverage was conducted by the International Harm Reduction Association (IHRA). In 2010 there were 82 countries or territories globally that implemented or tolerated NSP, and 70 countries that had MAT for PWID, i.e., five and seven more than in 2008, respectively. This shift is cause for optimism. However, reports from both the IHRA and the UN Reference Group stress that the coverage for PWID in countries currently implementing these interventions remains low, especially in high-burden countries. Several countries where a significant PWID population is present and HIV rates in that group are high—do not currently offer MAT (see Map 1.1).

Map 1.1   Global Availability of MAT, 2010

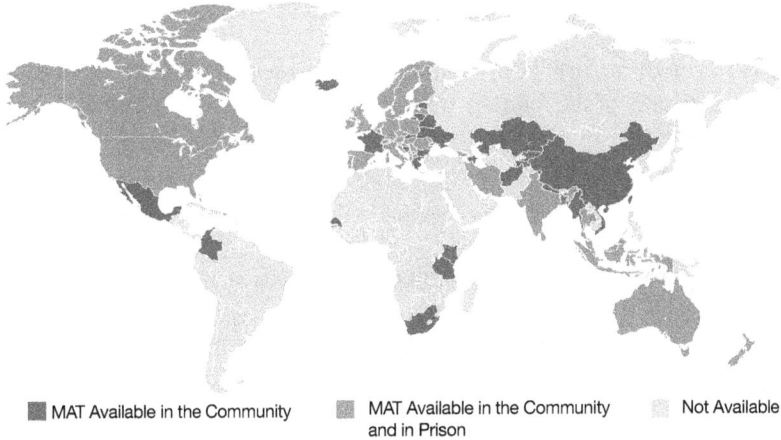

MAT Available in the Community   MAT Available in the Community   Not Available
and in Prison

Source: International Harm Reduction Association 2010.
Note: MAT = medically assisted therapy.

Box 1.2   Numbers Reached by Key Harm Reduction Interventions among PWID Globally: Sources of Data

The IDU Reference Group also provides data on the current number of sites and individuals reached for NSPs. Data are also available for MAT, other drug treatment, and HCT. The most recent substantive update of global data in this context was conducted in 2008. www.idureferencegroup.unsw.edu.au

In addition, the following sources can be consulted:

1. **Multi-country:** *HIV prevention, treatment, and care services for people who inject drugs: a systematic review of global, regional, and national coverage* (Mathers, Degenhardt et al. 2010)

2. **Multi-country:** *Global state of harm reduction 2010—key issues for broadening the response* (International Harm Reduction Association 2010)

3. **South and Southeast Asia:** *A situation update on HIV epidemics among people who inject drugs and national responses in South-East Asia Region.* (Sharma, Oppenheimer et al. 2009)

4. **Selected LMICs:** *Injection drug use, HIV and the current response in selected low-income and middle-income countries* (Bergenstrom and Abdul-Quader 2010)

Source: International Harm Reduction Association 2010.

Effects of the Four Key Interventions among PWID in the Context of the HIV Epidemic

We summarize the results from several recent reviews of studies related to the effectiveness of the four key interventions in reducing risky behaviors in the context of transmitting or acquiring HIV infection. We also review recent studies of the association between HIV outcomes (prevalence or incidence) and expanding the key interventions in isolation, especially NSP and MAT, or in combination. This review of available studies and evidence is an important element that contributes to the overall policy objectives.

We focus on the *direct effects* of these interventions. These are effects that are proximate to the risk of acquiring HIV infection in an individual who injects drugs. Direct effects at the individual level are connected. For example, there is some evidence that MAT can lead to a reduction in the total quantum of injecting drug use, which reduces the quantum of unsafe injecting episodes mechanically. However, unsafe injecting behavior can also be independently affected. For example, counseling as a part of a NSP can increase knowledge of risks when equipment is shared, as well as provide unused, sterile needles and syringes for the use of PWID. We consider the effect for which there is the most evidence from LMIC:

* Reduction in HIV incidence in PWID via reduction in risky behavior, sexual and injecting
  · Hence, reduced risk of infection in non-injecting partners (sexual) of PWID

In a community-level model, reducing HIV incidence among PWID and their non-injecting partners can be seen to reduce community levels of HIV transmission. This can occur where PWID are significant as a core or bridging group for HIV transmission into the general, lower risk population. Such reductions can depend on the local nature of sexual networks involving PWID, and their other risk behaviors, especially risky sexual contact. We consider this in our modeling approach, described in Chapter 2. The ability to model these effects is an advantage over more specific, PWID-focused models.

Excluded Effects in This Report

Other direct effects that can be considered are related to the morbidity & mortality averted among PWID who do not get infected with HIV. As the quantum of injecting drug use reduces, it may also be possible to estimate the number of overdose cases related to opioid drug use and the reduction therein as risky injecting drug use declines.

The reduction in HIV infection may contribute significantly to a reduced future morbidity and mortality burden in the PWID population. It may be possible to estimate these averted future HIV morbidity and mortality outcomes, and assess the averted costs of healthcare. However, due to lack of data on such outcomes and related costs in countries we consider as case studies, we did not extend the analysis to these health effects.

Our report also does not extend to the modeled results for two important yet difficult to estimate non-health outcomes from the four key interventions. These are considered 'indirect' in terms of the pathway to impact on the well-being of PWID. Such effects were discussed in recent reviews of harm reduction interventions among PWID (IOM 2007). Of these effects, and for our four key interventions, strong and consistent evidence is available for two key indirect effects: reduced criminality when this is related to drug use, and improved employment status of PWID as a result of the interventions.

Other effects include those stemming from medical comorbidities often observed within the HIV epidemic among PWID. There are also mental comorbidities, but data are even harder to find on these than the medical comorbidities for incidence, coverage of interventions against them, and the effectiveness of those interventions. Analysis can consider primarily certain medical comorbidities, specifically hepatitis-C virus (HCV), hepatitis-B virus (HBV), and tuberculosis (TB). We acknowledge the importance of bacterial infections. In addition to these co-morbidities, infective endocarditis is also a known complication and co-morbidity of injecting, the frequency of which has been best described in the developed world.

Evidence for NSP, MAT, and HCT Reducing Risk Behaviors among PWID

We did not conduct a systematic literature review for this report. There are recent comprehensive reviews of published studies involving the four key interventions, which we draw from to develop our summary below as well as to inform the modeling (Degenhardt, Mathers et al. 2010; Rhodes and Hedrich 2010). We also draw on an unpublished review of studies on the evidence from implementation of these interventions in LMIC settings. The sections below are also summarized in Box 1.3.

Evidence for the Effect of NSP on Risky Injecting Behaviors

There is strong and consistent evidence across LMIC for the effect of needle and syringe programs on risky injecting behaviors: sharing of injecting equipment, unsafe injection, and higher frequency of injection. Cumulative effect in this context should reduce the total number of risky injecting episodes, thereby reducing the risk of HIV acquisition.

Degenhardt et al. found references to the effect of NSP on risky injecting behavior in published studies including meta-analyses and high quality systematic reviews, or randomized control trials (Degenhardt, Mathers et al. 2010). Across these studies they rated the evidence for NSP reducing such risky behavior to be consistent and strong. A report sponsored by the European Monitoring Centre for Drugs and Drug Addiction (EMCDDA) considered three core reviews which in total report on 43 studies, 39 of them showing that NSPs reduce injecting risk behavior (Rhodes and Hedrich 2010).

Effectiveness in this context has been demonstrated in evaluations of programs. NSPs concentrate rarely only on the distribution of sterile needles and syringes. They may also provide education on HIV risk, referral to other services including HCT, as well as distribution of materials other than sterile needles or syringes, such as sterilizing liquid (bleach), cotton, sterile cookers, and condoms.

In the recent PEPFAR guidance related to "comprehensive HIV prevention for people who inject drugs" (PEPFAR 2010), the range of effect on risky injecting behavior is as high as a 60 percent reduction from a baseline. Specifically, the guidance notes that:

Consistent findings from evaluation studies of NSPs reveal that these programs increase the availability of sterile injection equipment, reduce the quantities of contaminated needles and other injection equipment in circulation, reduce the risk of new HIV infections, and result in referrals to other services such as ART for those eligible and HCT. Additionally, findings from a range of studies indicate that NSPs do not increase the numbers of persons who begin to inject drugs or increase the frequency of drug use. (PEPFAR 2010)

Evidence from the developed world (Europe and North America) forms a strong basis for studies included in the two reviews of reviews quoted above. In order to specifically extend the discussion to LMIC, we accessed an unpublished literature review for evidence.

In South Asia, a study of two north-eastern Indian states that implemented NSPs with funding from the Bill and Melinda Gates Foundation indicates that across successive surveys from 2006 to 2009, PWID practicing safer injecting practices increased from 31.8 percent to 37.6 percent (Mahapatra, Goswami et al. 2010). An evaluation of the needle exchange program in Dhaka from 2002 to 2004 using two successive behavioral surveillance surveys (BSS) suggested that PWID in areas with the intervention had safer injecting behaviors than those in non-intervention areas, though evidence was mixed on safer sexual practices of the PWID, specifically condom use in the last commercial sexual encounter (Azim, Hussein et al. 2005). There was a similar finding in an evaluation comparing intervention cities with NSPs operated by NGOs in Pakistan and other cities with PWID: more PWID in intervention cities (59 percent vs. 27 percent) reported always using a clean syringe. Average coverage of sterile syringes in intervention cities was 30 percent compared to 13 percent nationwide, though within a city coverage varied from 30 to 99 percent. Condom use at last commercial sex and HIV prevention knowledge also increased in intervention cities among PWID (Khan and Khan 2011).

In Eastern Europe, an observational cohort study of PWID in Georgia reporting on needle and syringe exchange suggested visible reductions in injection risk behaviors among clients of the program who had participated for at least three months. However, there was no significant change in sexual risk behaviors. In East Asia, a study reports the results of a prospective community-randomized prevention trial of a needle social marketing strategy. At baseline, needle sharing behaviors between control and intervention groups were similar. However, needle-sharing dropped significantly to 35.3 percent in the intervention community while remaining relatively stable in the control community (62.3 percent, p<0.001) (Pang, Hao et al. 2007).

Evidence for the Effect of MAT on Risky Injecting Behaviors

Medically Assisted Therapy, or MAT, for opioid dependence uses methadone, buprenorphine, or other combinations (including naltrexone) as an effective treatment to reduce need to inject opioids such as heroin. This is also called opioid substitution therapy or OST. We use the term MAT consistently in this report. When performed with methadone, MAT is often called Methadone Maintenance Therapy (MMT). Similarly, with buprenorphine, the intervention becomes Buprenorphine Maintenance Therapy or BMT.

According to the PEPFAR guidance, MAT has been demonstrated to be effective in reducing opioid dependence, reduce risk behaviors related to injection drug use, prevent HIV transmission, and improve PWID adherence to ART (PEPFAR 2010). The EMCDDA study considers three core reviews for the evidence of an effect of MAT on prevalence and frequency of injection; sharing of injecting equipment; and scores of drug-related risk. For our purposes, the second effect was of interest. Of the three core reviews surveyed, the Cochrane review, which is also the most recent review, concluded that MAT is associated with a significant reduction in the sharing of injecting equipment and injecting risk behavior (Gowing, Farrell et al. 2008). The Lancet paper also found that MAT is associated with a strong consistent negative effect on injecting risk behavior across the studies they reviewed (Degenhardt, Mathers et al. 2010).

Again, most of the evidence above derives from middle income and developed countries. Availability of MAT, and when available, its scale of coverage in LMIC has been poor, hence limiting the evidence base.

In South Asia, Armstrong et al. (2010) reported on outcomes in an NGO-run MAT program providing buprenorphine (BMT) to PWID in two north-eastern Indian states. The study finds that retention on treatment is a challenge, but in those that remained, there were statistically significant (p <0.05) improvements in frequency of needle sharing. In addition, there was a reduction in unsafe sex behaviors, as well as indirect effects reducing incidents of detention and in a range of quality of life measures (Armstrong, Kermode et al. 2010).

However, retention in BMT is still much higher than in programs that do not use an opioid agonist. For example, in Ukraine the initial scale-up of BMT demonstrated 75 percent retention at six months compared to the non-substitution drug based rehabilitation programs (33.3 percent). The initial evaluation of the Ukrainian experience suggests that the average addiction severity index—constructed from several indicators related to psychological and social well-being, including drug use—had improved significantly. Other data on BMT/MMT in Ukraine suggest MAT is able to achieve considerable decreases in injecting risk behaviors (p<0.01), with less pronounced reduction in sexual risk behaviors (Schaub, Chtenguelov et al. 2010).

In Asia, a pilot randomized clinical trial in Malaysia was implemented to evaluate whether the efficacy of office-based BMT, provided with limited counseling or oversight of medication adherence, was improved by the addition of individual drug counseling and abstinence-contingent take-home doses of buprenorphine. Two groups were assigned to either type of intervention. In both groups, the proportion of opioid-negative urine tests increased significantly over time (p<0.001), though the reductions were significant greater in those receiving enhanced services. The group receiving enhanced counseling and monitoring of adherence also achieved longer periods of consecutive abstinence from opiates (10.3 weeks vs. 7.8 weeks, p=0.154). Both groups receiving BMT services significantly reduced HIV risk behaviors during the treatment (p<0.05), and the difference between the groups was not statistically significant (Chawarski, Mazlan et al. 2008).

The aim of a longitudinal cohort study (Lawrinson, Ali et al. 2008) was to examine the effectiveness of MAT in lower income countries. Selected MAT sites in Asia (China, Indonesia, Thailand), Eastern Europe (Lithuania, Poland, Ukraine), Iran and Australia were included in the analysis with participants interviewed at treatment entry, three months, and then at six months. Treatment retention at six months averaged 70 percent, and all sites demonstrated significant and marked reductions in reported opioid use. The proportions reporting no heroin or other opioid use in the previous month at the six month point ranged from 69 percent in Thailand and 100 percent in China. Reduction in HIV-related risk behaviors (p<0.006) were reported, and psychological and social well-being improved over the course of the study.

In China, two different studies of MMT showed major declines in the proportion of clients injecting drugs and in the frequency of injection, covering a total of 1,710 clients (Pang, Hao et al. 2007; Qian, Hao et al. 2008). In both studies, the changes in use of opioids compared to baseline were significant. In one study, for those who had ever participated in MMT the odds related to using drugs, injecting drugs, and sharing needles or syringes were all significantly lower (Qian, Hao et al. 2008). There were also beneficial results in terms of reduction of unsafe sex practices. A separate study on MMT found an almost complete reduction in opioid use compared to the baseline by six months. None of the participants in MMT seroconverted to HIV or HCV positivity by six months (Institute of Medicine 2007).

Evidence for the Effect of HIV Counseling and Testing for PWID on Risk Behaviors for HIV

The *Lancet* paper (Degenhardt, Mathers et al. 2010) quotes a previous non-specific meta-analysis on the negative effect of HIV counseling and testing (HCT) on risk behaviors (Denison, O'Reilly et al. 2008). The meta-analysis does not cite evidence specific to PWID. There is limited evidence of an effect of HIV testing and counseling on risky injecting behaviors.

A recent WHO and UNAIDS guidance on voluntary HIV counseling and testing for PWID includes client-initiated and provider-initiated testing (WHO and UNODC 2009). The guidance suggests that reduction in sexual risk behaviors and HIV incidence are strongest only when counseling and testing is voluntary, and connected with access to risk-reduction materials (e.g., condoms) and information, and access to ART for those who are HIV-positive and need treatment.

In the context of LMIC, a study analyzed results from a project in Ukraine where a large number of PWID were tested for HIV (Booth, Lehman et al. 2009). The study compared prevention outreach using a more elaborate street-based method for reaching PWID with only the HCT intervention. Both interventions reduced injecting and sexual risk behaviors significantly. PWID who knew they were HIV-infected were more likely to practice safe sex compared to those who were unaware of their status or HIV-negative. Specifically, those who learned they were HIV-positive at baseline changed their sexual practices more than those who knew they were already infected, and those who were HIV-negative. This suggests, as for those not PWID, that HCT works to modify behaviors for those found HIV-positive that were unaware of their status, but not for those found HIV-negative.

A study examined the feasibility of NGO-provided voluntary HCT to PWID in southern China. The evaluation indicated that if the program was implemented properly, it would increase the participants' HIV-related knowledge and promote safer injecting and sexual practices

Overall, we find that evidence is stronger for an effect of HCT in reducing risky sexual behavior among PWID, rather than a reduction in risky injecting behavior.

Evidence for the Impact of NSP, MAT, ART, and HCT on HIV Incidence among PWID

The effect of interventions such as NSP and MAT on HIV incidence flows through the reduction in risky behaviors as suggested above. Studies using prospective cohort, case-control, ecological, mathematical modeling, and cross-sectional methodologies have attempted to demonstrate this effect.

The EMCDDA study looked at evidence from four reviews for the effect of NSPs on HIV incidence (and prevalence) which included 18 primary studies with HIV incidence outcomes (Rhodes and Hedrich 2010). These four reviews cover studies from the last two decades using the previously mentioned methods.

Of these, one review found mixed results of NSPs on incidence, which was related to the quality of the study or the design of the intervention, including effects such as selection bias in the participating PWID (IOM 2007). A review by Käll et al. (2007) concluded that the evidence for an effect of NSP on HIV outcomes was overrated (Käll, Hermansson et al. 2007). For studies with an HIV prevalence outcome, Käll et al. found that three longitudinal studies showed a negative association of NSP use and HIV seroprevalence, a finding matched by ecological studies which offer less robust evidence because they did not control for probably confounding effects.

In contrast, two other reviews found that there is evidence to support the effect of NSPs in reducing HIV incidence among PWID (Gibson, Flynn et al. 2001; Wodak and Cooney 2004). Overall, Degenhardt et al. (2010) conclude that the evidence from high-quality systematic reviews indicates that NSPs have a negative effect on HIV incidence, albeit with some inconsistent conclusions.

Mathematical modeling can simulate an epidemiological situation to allow for deeper analysis of the effect of interventions. A study analyzing the estimated impact of NSPs in Australia suggested that the annual distribution of 30 million sterile syringes in Australia would be able to control HIV transmission among

PWID at low levels. This effect should continue with the maintenance of the current programs. However, the study found that control of hepatitis-C virus (HCV) would be much harder to achieve (Kwon, Iversen et al. 2009).

For MAT, three reviews, including a Cochrane review from 2008 are quoted in the EMCDDA study. The reviews covered eight studies, of which two were randomized control trials and four cohort studies (Rhodes and Hedrich 2010). The conclusions from all reviews were consistent in that they found that continuous MAT was associated with lower rates of HIV seroconversion. In particular, one review concluded that the risk of HIV seroconversion was inversely related to the length of time in MAT (IOM 2007)[1].

There is recent evidence that ART outcomes for PWID are similar to non-PWID when they are similarly adherent to treatment even when the ART is the routine design and not 'directly observed'. A recent guidelines document summarizes the evidence in this context and suggests that early studies which showed poorer effects for ART in PWID covered interventions with selection bias, poor adherence support for the IDU, and mortality due to non-HIV related conditions (USAID, WHO et al. 2007). The document quotes recent evidence from 6,645 patients on ART across 51 centers in Europe that found response on ART to be similar between PWID and non-PWID, and a Canadian study of 1,522 PWID and non-PWID who had similar increases in CD4 t-cell counts on ART.

Fewer studies have considered combinations of interventions and the effect on HIV incidence. Wiessing et al. (2009) conducted a non-causal, ecological study of the association between the availability and coverage of MAT and NSP in the European Union and five middle- and high-income countries including Ukraine. Countries with greater provision of both prevention measures in 2000 to 2004 had lower incidence of diagnosed HIV infection among PWID in 2005 to 2006 (Wiessing, Likatavicius et al. 2009).

Of particular interest to us are studies based on mathematical models attempting to attribute impact on HIV incidence from combination prevention, i.e., with the key harm reduction interventions as well as structural and community interventions, if present.

The modeling of reduction in injecting risk behaviors to a reduction in risk of HIV infection involves several complexities. The relation between reductions in frequency of sharing needles and HIV transmission is complex, based on modeling of PWID populations in Russia and London (Degenhardt, Mathers et al. 2010). Indeed if infection risk in a community is sufficiently high due to prevailing HIV positivity levels and sexual practices, then eliminating risky injecting behaviors may not lead to major declines in levels of infection—a phenomenon termed "risk redundancy".

A recent global study used point estimates of reduction in an individual's HIV infection risk per unit time (60 percent for MAT, 40 percent for NSP, and 90 percent for ART) to suggest that if coverage in a range of global PWID-based epidemics were raised, there would be significant effects on HIV incidence (Degenhardt, Mathers et al. 2010). These effects are modeled via the channel of reduced injecting risk behaviors as well as reduced viral load among PWID as a result of being on ART. Sexual risk reduction and effect on transmission were not modeled. If at the end of five years the coverage levels among PWID for MAT plus NSP were 51 percent, the median estimate of relative reduction in HIV incidence over five years was nearly 20 percent. Adding ART at 50 percent coverage among eligible PWID would increase the reduction in HIV incidence to nearly 35 percent from the baseline.

Overall, the literature on the linkage between the key interventions with PWID and HIV outcomes is well-developed in the context of developed countries and has been recently reviewed elsewhere (Beyrer, Malinows-ka-Sempruch et al. 2010a; Degenhardt, Mathers et al. 2010; Beyrer 2011a). However, given the differences in the contexts of injecting drug use it would be preferable to review studies analyzing impact on incidence in LMIC.

From such LMIC, there are only a few studies with HIV prevalence or incidence outcomes. One study looked at the NSPs in Yunnan, China that began operation in 2002 in response to the HIV epidemic among PWID. The authors used a mathematical model to estimate the population benefits in terms of infections averted and the cost-effectiveness of the NSP. It is estimated that the NSP in Yunnan averted approximately 16 to 20 percent (5,200 to 7,500) of the expected HIV cases and led to gains of 1,300 to 1,900 DALYs. The total of US$1.04 million spent on NSP from 2002–08 yielded a cost-saving of US$1.38–$1.97 million via the averted costs of prevention, care, and patient management (Lei, Lorraine et al.).

A study in Bangladesh utilized a mathematical transmission model to estimate the impact of the CARE-Shakti harm reduction intervention for PWID in Dhaka (Azim, Hussein et al. 2005). The national HIV surveillance data among PWID over 2000–2002 were compared to results from a dynamic mathematical model. The model was used to predict the impact of the NSP intervention on HIV transmission among PWID. The results indicated that the NSP may have reduced the incidence of HIV among PWID by 90 percent (95 percent CI: 74–94 percent) after the duration of the intervention, holding the HIV prevalence at 10 percent (95 percent CI: 4–19 percent). In the absence of the intervention, the model predicted that the HIV prevalence would be 42 percent (95 percent CI: 30–47 percent).

Table 1.2   Summary of Evidence for NSP, MAT, and HCT in Reducing Risk Behaviors and HIV Incidence among PWID in LMIC

Study	Country	Type of Study	Intervention	Conclusion
A. Evidence for NSP, MAT, and HCT in reducing risk behaviors among PWID				
Degenhardt, Mathers et al. 2010	Multi-country	Review of reviews	NSP	Strong and consistent evidence for the effect of NSPs in reducing various risky injecting behaviors
Rhodes and Hedrich 2010	Multi-country	Review of reviews	NSP	39 of 43 studies included in 3 core reviews found that NSPs reduce risky injecting behaviors
Mahapatra, Goswami et al. 2010	India	Observational (cross-section)	NSP	Proportion of PWID practicing safer injecting practices increased in intervention districts from 31.8% to 37.6%
Azim, Hussein et al. 2005	Bangladesh	Observational (cross-section)	NSP	PWID in intervention areas had safer injecting behaviors than in non-intervention areas.
Khan and Khan 2011	Pakistan	Observational (cross-section)	NSP	More PWID in intervention vs. non-intervention cities (59% vs. 27%) reported always using a clean syringe; condom use at last commercial sex also increased in intervention cities among PWID
Otiashvili, Gambashidze et al. 2006	Georgia	Observational (cohort study)	NSP	Reduction in risky injecting behaviors for clients in the program for at least three months. No significant change in sexual risk behavior.
Wu, Luo et al. 2007	PR of China	Community-randomized trial	NSP	Needle sharing behaviors dropped from 68.4% to 35.3% in the intervention group, and remained relatively stable in the control (p<0.001)
Gowing, Farrell et al. 2008	Multi-country	Systematic review	MAT	MAT is associated with a significant reduction in the sharing of injecting equipment and injecting risk behaviors
Armstrong, Kermode et al. 2010	India	Observational (cohort study)	MAT	Statistically significant (p=0.05) improvements were observed in relation to needle sharing and unsafe sex
Schaub, Chtenguelov et al. 2010	Ukraine	Observational (cohort study)	MAT	Considerable decreases in injecting risk behaviors (p<0.01), with less pronounced reduction in sexual risk behaviors

(Continued next page)

Table 1.2 *(continued)*

Study	Country	Type of Study	Intervention	Conclusion
Chawarski, Mazlan et al. 2008	Malaysia	Randomized trial	MAT	Proportion of opioid-negative urine tests increased significantly (p<0.001), and groups significantly reduced HIV risk behaviors (p<0.05)
Lawrinson, Ali et al. 2008	Set of LMIC	Longitudinal cohort study	MAT	Proportions reporting no opioid use in the previous month at the six month point ranged from 69% in Thailand to 100% in China.
Qian, Hao et al. 2008	PR of China	Observational (survey)	MAT	Those currently enrolled in methadone maintenance had lower risk of using and injecting drugs than those who were no longer receiving methadone
Pang, Hao et al. 2007	PR of China	Observational (cohort study)	MAT	Among clients, frequency of injection in the past month had reduced from 90 times per month to twice per month over 12 months of enrolment
Booth, Lehman et al. 2009	Ukraine	Quasi-experimental	HCT	PWID who first learned that they were infected at baseline changed their safe sex practices significantly more than those who already knew and those HIV-negative.
B. Evidence for the impact of NSP, MAT, ART, and HCT on HIV incidence among PWID				
Mathers, Degenhardt et al. 2010	Multi-country	Review of reviews	NSP	Evidence from high-quality systematic reviews indicates that NSPs have a negative effect on HIV incidence, albeit with some inconsistent conclusions
Tilson, Aramrattana et al. 2007	Multi-country	Systematic review	NSP	The evidence of the effectiveness of NSPs in reducing HIV prevalence is considered modest based on the weakness of the included study designs
Käll, Hermansson et al. 2007	Multi-country	Systematic review	NSP	[for HIV prevalence] three longitudinal studies showed a negative association between NSP coverage and HIV prevalence, matched by ecological studies
Wodak and Cooney 2004	Multi-country	Systematic review	NSP	There is compelling evidence that increasing the availability and utilization of sterile injecting equipment by PWID reduces HIV infection substantially

Table 1.2 *(continued)*

Study	Country	Type of Study	Intervention	Conclusion
Kwon, Iversen et al. 2009	Australia	Mathematical modeling	NSP	Annual distribution of 30 million sterile syringes would be able to control HIV transmission among PWID at low levels
Rhodes and Hedrich 2010	Multi-country	Review of reviews	MAT	Evidence from 2 randomized control trials and four cohort studies suggests that continuous MAT was associated with lower rates of HIV seroconversion. Risk of HIV seroconversion is inversely related to the length of time in MAT
USAID, WHO et al. 2007	Multi-country	Non-systematic review	ART	Based on 6,645 patients on ART in 51 centers in Europe; 1,522 PWID in Canada–response on ART for PWID is similar to non–PWID
Wiessing, Likatavi-cius et al. 2009	Multi-country (incl. Ukraine)	Ecological analysis	MAT, NSP	Countries with higher provision of both interventions over 2000 to 2004 had lower incidence of HIV among PWID in 2005 to 2006
Degenhardt, Mathers et al. 2010	Global	Mathematical modeling	MAT, NSP, ART	If coverage of these interventions was raised in a range of global PWID-based epidemics, there would be significant decreases in HIV incidence
Lei, Lorraine et al. 2011	PR of China	Mathematical modeling	NSP	NSP in Yunnan province averted approximately 16-20% of the expected HIV cases and led to gains of 1,300 to 1,900 DALYs
Foss, Watts et al. 2007	Bangladesh	Mathematical modeling	NSP	NSP may have reduced the incidence of HIV among PWID by 90%, resulting in HIV prevalence of 10% instead of 42% if the intervention had not occurred
VAHC, UNAIDS et al. 2010	Vietnam	Mathematical modeling	NSP	In 7 provinces, harm reduction provinces may have averted between 2% to 56% of infections in PWID, depending on the level of program coverage
Alistar, Owens et al. 2011	Ukraine	Mathematical modeling	ART, MAT	A dual ART-MAT strategy with 80% ART coverage and 25% MAT coverage was able to avert 8,300 HIV infections versus no intervention

Source: Authors.
Note: ART = antiretroviral therapy; HCT = HIV counseling and testing; MAT = medically assisted theapy; NSP = needle and syringe program.

In Vietnam, the World Bank and UNAIDS supported an evaluation of the country's harm reduction strategy. The study had several levels of findings. At the ecological analysis level, in 12 of the 19 provinces with data, high levels of per capita needle-syringe distribution (i.e., more than 100 needle-syringes per PWID) corresponded with a stable or declining HIV prevalence trend among PWID. From a modeling analysis incorporated in the same report, the results suggest that in seven provinces, harm reduction programs averted between 2 percent to 56 percent of infections in PWID, depending on the level of program coverage. The prevention activities among PWID and female sex workers (FSW) in Vietnam also interrupt other chains of transmission, leading to reduction in secondary infections (VAHC, UNAIDS et al. 2010).

Returning to Ukraine, another dynamic compartmental mathematical model found that scaling up ART to 80 percent coverage and MAT to 25 percent coverage was able to avert 8,300 infections versus no intervention. Comparing the dual ART-MAT strategy to a MAT-only strategy meant the addition of 105,000 QALYs at US$1,120/QALY gained. A MAT-only strategy was the most cost-effective, reducing infections by 4,700 and adding 76,000 QALYs compared with no intervention, at US$530/QALY gained (Alistar, Owens et al. 2011)

The studies above suggest compelling evidence for countries with high levels of HIV prevalence among PWID to increase the coverage of the four key interventions, which will yield significant returns in reduced HIV incidence and hence reduced levels of future morbidity, mortality, and healthcare costs. Specific evidence from countries is available and has been reviewed. Such analyses can be improved by modeling connections with community levels of incidence, and incorporation of reductions in sexual transmission risk among PWID.

Table 1.2 summarizes the literature review in the sections above. We did not formally grade the quality of evidence from these studies.

Organization of this Report

Chapter 1 conducted a brief global situation assessment of harm reduction for PWID and a review of reviews on the effectiveness of NSP, MAT, HCT, and ART for PWID in the context of HIV prevention. In conducting our review of effectiveness, we identified a critical lack of information in terms of studies on the effect of the interventions and HIV outcomes in developing countries. We highlight the importance of epidemiological context as well as the differences in interpretation of the results of previous studies that are mostly derived from the developed world. An important aspect of providing economic evidence for increased advocacy in LMIC is to conduct case studies across several different LMIC contexts.

Chapter 2 provides more information on our methodology for the rest of this report, including the selection criteria for case studies. The chapter discusses the modeling strategy for the cases and the type of data used. The chapter considers the methodological implications of modeling effects of key interventions in combination rather than in isolation, given the type of evidence available.

Chapters 3 to 6 of this report are individual case studies of four different LMIC countries with differing epidemics of HIV among PWID. In each case study, we provide an overall epidemiological overview that highlights key recent developments in the epidemic and in the country's response. We conduct a model-based analysis of the effect of scaling-up the four key interventions in combination.

We hope that the case studies with their epidemic overviews and model-based analyses of the effect of expanding coverage of key interventions among PWID provide compelling evidence for renewed investment. Chapter 7 helps to reinforce this with an overall discussion of the results across the case studies and their implications for global policy related to scale-up of key harm reduction interventions among PWID.

Note

1. Since the time of this research, a global review of published and unpublished findings has been published, estimating an approximate 54% reduction in risk for HIV transmission associated with use of MAT (Macarthur et al. 2012).

CHAPTER 2

Methodology

Country Case Studies

In discussion with the World Bank and partners, the study team identified an initial group of countries that represented a diverse selection across PWID-HIV epidemic contexts. These countries were: Ukraine, Kenya, Thailand, Argentina, and Pakistan. Given the availability of data and the engagement of in-country partners, all of the case studies except Argentina were selected for analysis. These country case studies address a range of PWID population sizes, types of drug use, and different prevailing HIV epidemic contexts. They represent a sub-Saharan epidemic context (Kenya), Eastern Europe and its established HIV epidemics among PWID (Ukraine), South Asia and its developing epidemics among PWID (Pakistan), and Southeast Asia with its mature HIV epidemics among PWID (Thailand).

Research Questions

For each case study, the modeled time period for expansion of coverage of the four key interventions was 2012 to 2015, and the base year was 2011. The following research questions were used for the modeling component of each case study. They apply a concept of unmet need, discussed further:

a. What is the impact on HIV incidence of implementing the key interventions at a level of coverage eliminating a substantial portion of the unmet need?

b. What is the cost of expanding the key interventions to eliminate the unmet need? Based on direct effects, what is the cost-effectiveness of the expansion?

c. What is the uncertainty around costing and cost-effectiveness results for implementation of the four key interventions and how can these uncertainties best be addressed?

Unmet Need

The current PWID population size and HIV prevalence, as well as the estimated current coverage of the four key interventions, are inputs into a projection of the required expansion of interventions, i.e., the required or desired coverage. In this process, the knowledge of what is feasible is important–pragmatic considerations may prevent us from modeling an expansion to 'high' levels of coverage among PWID (see Table 2.1) within the timeframe of modeling, i.e., up to 2015 from the base, 2011.

Table 2.1   Target Coverage Levels, from the Technical Guide

	NSP: percentage of PWID regularly reached by NSP	MAT: percentage of opioid-dependent people on MAT at census date	HCT: percentage of PWID who received an HIV test in past 12 mo. and know the results	ART: percentage of eligible HIV-positive PWID receiving ART
Low	≤20%	≤20%	≤40%	≤25%
Medium	>20–≤60%	>20–≤ 40%	>40–≤ 75%	>25–≤75%
High	>60%	>40%	>75%	>75%

Source: WHO, UNODC et al. 2009.
Note: ART = antiretroviral therapy; HCT = HIV counseling and testing; MAT = medically assisted therapy; NSP = needle and syringe program.

The comparison of the expanded levels of coverage, when compared with the levels of coverage for key interventions based on a continuation of current trends, serves to illustrate the "unmet need" (Figure 2.1).

Introduction to the Modeling Methodology

We use the Goals mathematical model to conduct the analysis. This model has been utilized in multiple studies over the last decade, including for a similar report on MSM (Beyrer, Wirtz et al. 2011). Goals is an integrated module within the Spectrum suite of models (Futures Institute 2012). It reads demographic and epidemic projections from other Spectrum modules, such as demographic projections and the numbers related to the evolution of the HIV epidemic over time in terms of individuals in various behavioral risk groups, CD4 t-cell bands, and hence the numbers of adults needing antiretroviral treatment based on country guidelines.

Figure 2.1   Hypothetical "Unmet Need"—Difference between Baseline and Expanded Scenarios (NSP)

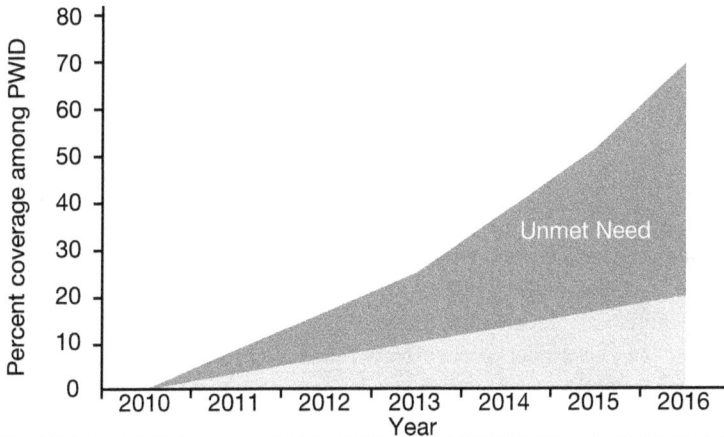

	2010	2011	2012	2013	2014	2015	2016
Expanded	0	5	10	15	25	35	50
Baseline	0	3.33	6.67	10	13.33	16.67	20

Source: Authors.
Note: NSP = needle and syringe program.

Goals simulates an HIV epidemic by estimating the number of new HIV infections occurring in various population risk groups according to their behaviors and the coverage and effectiveness of interventions. The population groups are divided into: low, medium and high-risk heterosexuals; PWID; and men who have sex with men (MSM). Users of the model specify the population size for each group and the characteristics of the expected risk behavior. Changes to future behavior are modeled based on changes in interventions which change the behavior of the populations and ultimately the number of new infections. Baseline coverage levels for interventions are usually based on country level reporting, and incorporated in percentage coverage terms.

As mentioned, Spectrum helps to rigorously specify demographic and epidemiological assumptions for each country case. The integrated demographic projection platform, which is routinely calibrated in-country by government and technical partners, is a starting point for medium- and long-term projections of HIV epidemics. The Spectrum suite has been widely used in Asia, Africa, and Eastern Europe. Its use for this proposed activity provides continuity for country stakeholders and partners. It has also been used recently to inform the World Bank's Global HIV/AIDS Program's (GHAP) research agenda (Table 2.2).

Table 2.2   Recent Use of Goals for World Bank GHAP Analytical Projects

	Global HIV epidemics among MSM	Global HIV epidemics among FSW	Global HIV epidemics among PWID (IDU)
Modeled countries	Kenya, Peru, Thailand, Ukraine	Kenya, Cambodia, Brazil, Russian Fed.	Kenya, Ukraine, Thailand, Pakistan

Source: Authors.
Note: FSW = female sex worker; IDU = injecting drug user; MSM = men who have sex with men.

Modeling HIV Epidemics among PWID in the Goals Model

The Goals model is well situated to estimate the direct effect of reduced HIV incidence from expanding NSP and MAT interventions among PWID; based upon the potential reduction in frequency of needle sharing. If evidence is available, it can also incorporate effects based on a reduction in the number of needle sharing partners and in future versions of the model, in the quantum of injecting drug use. We discuss these effects in the context of the "Goals Impact Matrix" further below.

In addition to these two harm reduction interventions, Goals can incorporate the effects of HCT for PWID as per the evidence. As discussed in Chapter 1, we expect an effect from increasing coverage of voluntary HCT among PWID on unsafe sexual behavior, but not on unsafe injecting behavior.

For ART, Goals models the reduction in possibility of HIV transmission during unsafe sexual contact, produced from the reduced viral load from receiving and being adherent to antiretroviral drug treatment. Goals does not assume or involve any parameters linked to a reduction in the possibility of HIV transmission (i.e., parenteral transmission) related to unsafe injecting behavior when PWID receive ART.

Any decline in HIV incidence which occurs among PWID, their sexual partners, and in the wider community level from expansion of interventions can be quantitatively estimated by comparing different Goals projections (e.g., a baseline projection or scenario versus one with expansion of key interventions).

Epidemiological and Behavioral Inputs Related to PWID Required in Goals Modeling

Besides the coverage of behavioral interventions and biomedical interventions, the Goals model also requires inputs related to levels of the risky behaviors in the risk groups present in the population. Goals, utilizes the following time-invariant parameters in creating its projections for PWID. These are similar to those for all other risk groups, except for [#]3:

1. Percent of adult population 15–49 (male) that corresponds to male PWID

2. Percent of adult population 15–49 (female) that corresponds to female PWID

3. Percent of PWID sharing needles, average for both male and female

4. Percent of exits from the risk group replaced by increased recruitment (default is 100%)

The following time-variant value is needed in order to calibrate the scale-up of MAT for opioid injectors:

5. Percentage of PWID injecting opiates vs. non-opiates (e.g., stimulants)

The following are entered for as many years as available. These values are used only for model fitting purposes, i.e., to compare with the prevalence curve estimated within Goals for male and female PWID:

6. HIV prevalence among PWID, disaggregated by gender

Table 2.3   Certain Behavioral Inputs Needed for Goals Modeling Related to PWID

Input	Across years	Definition
Average duration of behavior (years): male PWID	Fixed	Number of years the average PWID injects drugs, end to end
Average duration of behavior (years): female PWID	Fixed	
Force of infection: male PWID (value from 0 to 1)	Variable	Number of new infections ÷ (number of susceptible exposed × average duration of exposure)
Force of infection: female PWID (value from 0 to 1)	Variable	
Percent of PWID sharing needles	Variable	Denominator: all PWID
Percent married, male PWID	Fixed	This can include those in other union with sexual contact

Source: Authors.

Cost Inputs Required in Goals Modeling

Goals requires the unit costs for several types of interventions and healthcare delivery elements within the HIV program. Costs can be varied from year to year, in order to represent economies of scale, or expected changes to program characteristics or target population. Costs are variable across the years of the projection. They can also be entered for prior years, but those costs will not enter the cost calculation. Estimating the PWID unit costs (e.g., cost per PWID covered with NSP, cost per PWID covered with MAT) require calculations outside Goals, as these costs are exogenous to the model. Some of the critical unit costs are discussed in Table 2.4 below.

Table 2.4   PWID-Specific Unit Cost of Interventions per Year (Unless Specified)

Unit Cost	PWID Specific?	Considerations
Adult ART per person	Non-specific	Costs for ART per person year are the same across groups.
HCT cost per PWID per test	Specific	Cost of HCT is estimated specifically for PWID.
NSP cost per PWID	Specific	This cost can be an average from current NSP in the country; coverage can be used to derive a cost curve.
MAT cost per PWID	Specific	Costs can be weighted averages across methadone and buprenorphine maintenance programs; use a cost curve.

Source: Authors.
Note: ART = antiretroviral therapy; HCT = HIV counseling and testing; MAT = medically assisted therapy; NSP = needle and syringe program.

Goals estimates costs in constant US dollars. The process of estimating unit costs will include identification of categories of resources used by the intervention package and determining the denominator appropriate to estimate the unit cost (coverage). Data utilized in estimating intervention cost include such items as: 1) costs of all commodities used in the intervention; 2) labor costs for intervention workers; 3) promotional and advertising costs; 4) average time clients spent with intervention; 5) rent; 6) maintenance; 7) incentives to participants; 8) volunteer activities; 9) user fees; 10) value of donated goods and services; and 11) other relevant costs.

Goals Impact Matrix

In Goals an "impact matrix" translates coverage of key behavioral and PWID interventions into reductions in certain behaviors from their baseline value. It does not cover effects of ART on the biological risk of transmitting or acquiring

HIV infection, nor does it have any other biomedical intervention. Those effects are managed elsewhere. However, it does include the PWID-specific interventions NSP and MAT, and has a row to insert another PWID intervention. We utilize this available row to capture HCT for PWID.

The default matrix provided with Goals contains parameters which are derived from periodically updated literature review across the following databases: EMBASE, Biosis, SciSearch, and SIGLE. In addition, the literature search encompasses reports from UNAIDS, DFID, FHI, Horizons Project, and Futures Group. It has been updated continuously every year since 2001, with the most recent update of the default matrix in September 2011. The methodology and inclusion/exclusion criteria are:

- The HIV/AIDS related intervention is from a developing country (Asia, Latin America, Africa)
- Provides pre-/post-intervention measures of the key variable
- Provides at least one useful endpoint (e.g., condom use, number of sexual partners, age at first sex, contacts with sex workers, etc.)
- Contains non-English reports for PWID interventions, otherwise English language studies

The impact matrix currently contains the results of reviewing 141 studies (12 percent of which were randomized control trials, 16 percent were quasi-experimental and 32 percent longitudinal). Studies from sub-Saharan Africa predominate (41 percent), followed by Asia (34 percent). The impact matrix values used in our modeling are discussed below, after we introduce the scenarios used for each case study.

Outputs and Limitations of Goals

From Goals, we can extract a number of outcomes for each case study, including numbers of new infections, HIV prevalence, and AIDS deaths in different modeling scenarios. These scenarios are described in the next section. Each modeling output is generated for both PWID and for the population as a whole in order to reflect the scale to which the PWID population contributes to the epidemic. Goals will also calculate the total cost of the scale-up of interventions.

Goals can be used to estimate the cost per infection averted for the range of interventions included in the national response. When two scenarios (projections) are conducted for a case study, Goals has a functionality to allow quantitative comparisons between the scenarios. This comparison involves the computation of the incremental cost-effectiveness per infection averted.

The scenarios considered for this activity will differ only to the extent of the increase in the coverage of NSP, MAT, HCT, and ART for PWID. Therefore, the difference in costs of service delivery over the projection period will primarily derive from these programs. A minor element of the cost differential may derive from secondary effects such as changes to community-level incidence of HIV and hence change in future need for treatment).

Goals is limited in being unable to identify the contribution to overall reductions in mortality and incidence from expansion of ART in a specific population group. In the current Goals model set-up, the user is only able to specify coverage of ART overall, not in specific groups. ART coverage is by default 'allocated' to the different population groups (low/medium/high-risk heterosexuals, MSM, etc.) based on their proportional size in the adult population. We discuss a response to this limitation in the next section.

Modeling the Effect of Scaling Up the Four Key Harm Reduction Interventions

Scenarios Used in Each Case Study

In each country case study, we consider three types of scenarios for Goals modeling:

- **Status Quo:** No change in the coverage of ART, NSP, MAT, or HCT for PWID over the years 2011–2015. Coverage of ART among adults 15–49 is maintained at the level achieved in 2011.

- **Baseline:** In this scenario the increase from levels of coverage of NSP, MAT, and HCT for PWID from the base year of 2011 across the period 2012–2015 is as per existing national plans. This coverage over 2012–2015 may be the same as the level in 2011 if we foresee no meaningful expansion or if plans do not call for increase. Using existing planned coverage may involve non-provision of one or more of the interventions in years 2012–2015. In this scenario, ART coverage increases every year over 2012–2015 based on the country's current scale-up plan for adult treatment. Related data are available from country-level sources or filed with UNAIDS. In most countries, even in the developed world, PWID have less than proportionate access to ART, i.e., the proportion of PWID on ART is less than the proportion of HIV-positive PWID in all HIV-positive adults (USAID, WHO et al. 2007). In contrast, the Baseline scenario assumes that PWID have proportionate access to ART slots as the intervention scales up, though the proportion used for allocation will be PWID as a proportion of all adults, 15–49 years. This allocation represents a major increase in the access to and utilization of life-saving treatment in this marginalized group, as well as a significant effect on the risk of HIV transmission through sexual contact among PWID and partners.

- **Expansion:** This scenario involves a scale-up of levels of provision of NSP, MAT, and HCT for PWID beyond national plans. The ranges for scale-up of each intervention used are from the WHO/UNODC/UNAIDS Technical Guide (see Table 2.1). The specific value used from the guideline range (whether the "Low", "Medium" or "High" range) is dictated by evaluating the country's current levels of provision and making a pragmatic yet ambitious judgment. For example, if a country is at zero or negligible coverage in 2011, then selecting a value for the scale reached in 2015 from the "Low" range of the guidelines may be appropriate.

Modeled Impact of Levels of Coverage of Key Interventions on PWID Risk Behaviors

Optimistic Impact: Table 2.5 describes an impact matrix we constructed for this report that uses point estimates from the upper range for effects of the three PWID interventions: NSP, MAT, and HCT. The values are suggested by the sources from the literature from the developed world, and are aspirational for LMIC contexts. The interpretation is of effects from high-quality interventions implemented in LMIC.

Table 2.5   Optimistic Impact Matrix of Three Key Harm Reduction Interventions for PWID

Intervention	Reduction in condom non-use: PWID	Reduction in number of sexual partners: PWID	Reduction in proportion of PWID sharing needles	Reduction in number of sharing partners: PWID
HCT	-24.2%	-	-	-
NSP	-42.0%	-1.2%	-33.8%	-
MAT	-	-	-95.7%	-

Source: Authors.
Note: - = not available; ART = antiretroviral therapy; HCT = HIV counseling and testing; MAT = medically assisted therapy; NSP = needle and syringe program.

Conservative Impact: Table 2.6 describes an impact matrix supplied as default with the Goals model. The values are suggested by sources from the literature that draw from LMIC experience, and reflect standard, guidelines-based implementation of the intervention, though not at quality seen in developed country contexts. The interpretation is of implementation at the beginning of a learning curve.

Table 2.6   Conservative Impact Matrix of Three Key Harm Reduction Interventions for PWID

Intervention	Reduction in condom non-use: PWID	Reduction in number of sexual partners: PWID	Reduction in proportion of PWID sharing needles	Reduction in number of sharing partners: PWID
HCT	-	-	-	-
NSP	-27.0%	-1.2%	-27.1%	-
MAT	-	-	-63.0%	-

Source: Authors.
Note: - = not available; ART = antiretroviral therapy; HCT = HIV counseling and testing; MAT = medically assisted therapy; NSP = needle and syringe program.

The impact matrices above show the impact of the intervention on the level of the risk behavior in the covered population, in the form of a percentage reduction of the behavior from its baseline value specified elsewhere in Goals. A blank cell in the impact matrix means no effect. The impact matrices above relate only to the proportion of a population that is covered by interventions. The reductions in levels of risk behaviors have an incidence response based on previously set parameters in the model controlling probability of transmission or acquisition of HIV infection during risky sexual or injecting episodes.

Both the optimistic and conservative matrices posit no effect of HCT on any of the PWID behaviors, as discussed in Chapter 1. They also posit that there are no effects on the number of sharing partners, just on the proportion who actually indulge in sharing. This is driven by a lack of evidence for the former effect.

It is difficult to compare the values above to the modeled results from other studies such as Alistar et al. for Ukraine (2011), due to difference in the methodology. However, the methods here are comparable to other modeling studies. Of these, we can point to the calculation exercise in a recent global study (Degenhardt et al., 2010) which uses point estimates of reduction in an individual's HIV infection risk per unit time (60 percent for MAT, 40 percent for NSP) to suggest that if coverage in a range of global PWID-based epidemics were raised, there would be significant effects on HIV incidence.[1]

Though it is not a part of the impact matrix, which concerns mostly behavioral effects, we assume that the provision of ART has the same preventive benefit among PWID as in other populations. This is via reduced viral load in successful therapy. We assume an 87 percent reduction in infectiousness when responding on ART compared to the asymptomatic stage of HIV disease with no ART. Specifically, for PWID, there is the issue of linkage between ART and MAT, which we discuss below.

Consideration of the Variable Effect of Interventions in Isolation and in Combination

The two impact matrices represent sensitivity analysis around the parameters of effect on risk behaviors. Using both of these impact matrices establishes a 'high / low' sensitivity check on the effects we are modeling from interventions to behaviors. We conducted explicit uncertainty analysis to further explore the values in the impact matrix. This is useful since we do not know the true population-level effect of these interventions, and because much of our knowledge on effectiveness comes from particular geographies, producing some limits to generalizability.

A separate issue to be explored in sensitivity or uncertainty analysis concerns the design of Goals. As a default Goals models the effect of interventions acting independently on the behavior noted in the impact matrix. Theoretically, there may be synergy and dependency issues around the interventions (Figure 2.2).

Figure 2.2   Pathways of Synergy and Dependence across the Four Key Harm Reduction Interventions

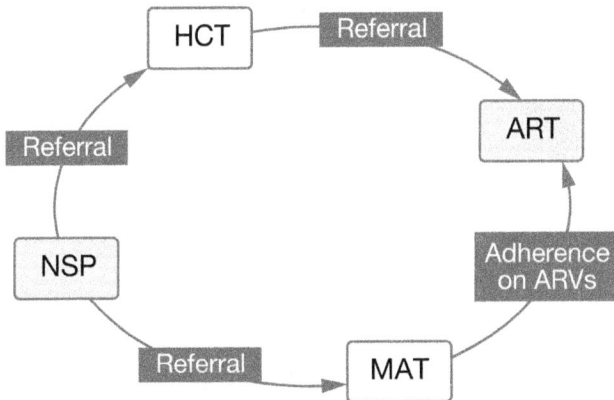

Source: Authors.
Note: ART = antiretroviral therapy; ARV = antiretroviral; HCT = HIV counseling and testing; MAT = medically assisted therapy; NSP = needle and syringe program.

We note that the current WHO guidelines do not make abstinence from injecting drug use mandatory for starting ART. A study from Brazil estimated adherence rates of 69 percent among low-income PWID on ART, without the use of MAT. A study from France of PWID with both MAT (buprenorphine) and ART showed 78 percent adherence to the latter (Coalition ARV4IDUs 2004). However, we acknowledge the problematic adherence to ART issues in those who are not abstaining from active drug use; this points to the synergies of participating in MAT. We also think that recidivism in MAT should be considered in terms of its implication on simultaneous ART. Pharmacological interactions between methadone and various antiretrovirals have been examined but need to be understood in terms of effect on patient management, behaviors, and costs.

There may well also be an issue of redundancy if there is one really efficacious intervention with PWID that should or can be done first. In the "Conservative" matrix (Table 2.6), there is no such magic bullet intervention. In the "Optimistic" matrix (Table 2.5), one could argue that MAT appears highly efficacious in reducing needle sharing behaviors, and hence deserves priority scale-up within the context of harm reduction for PWID. However, given an emphasis on providing combinations of interventions to maximize multi-dimensional impact among PWID (e.g., including reduction in overdose), we do not test a scenario with only MAT in isolation.

A problem we encounter in acting on the knowledge of synergies is that we have no quantitative estimate of what this synergy 'pays off' in terms of effects. Our effect parameters (Tables 2.5 and 2.6) are derived from the literature that has mostly evaluated these interventions in isolation, measuring the observed change in the behavior of interest. Till such studies of the synergistic effect are conducted, we have no quantitative basis for modeling synergy.

However, we can hypothesize that the effect is higher if synergies are present. In other words, the Optimistic matrix represents the higher end of effects seen from higher-quality, synergistic interventions. Whether the matrix represents the effect of higher quality vs. greater synergy is difficult to separate.

Optimistic Impact Matrix:
- World with higher stand-alone effects from the scale-up of NSP, HCT, and MAT interventions. Assumption is that there are synergies as in Figure 2.2, or quality of implementation is high

Conservative Impact Matrix:
- World with lower stand-alone effects on behaviors from the scale-up of NSP, HCT and MAT interventions. Assumption is that there are no synergies as suggested in the diagram

Overall, the sensitivity analysis suggests the following scenarios to run for each case study:

Status Quo	+	Conservative Impact Matrix	1. Status Quo Scenario
Baseline Scenario	+	Conservative Impact Matrix	2. Baseline Scenario
Expansion Scenario	+	Conservative Impact Matrix	3. Expansion Conservative Scenario
		Optimistic Impact Matrix	4. Expansion Optimistic Scenario

Uncertainty Analysis

Since we are not sure about the generalizability of the point estimates of the stand-alone effects, or their measurement error, we can also conduct uncertainty analysis. The following parameters were considered for the uncertainty analysis: values in the impact matrix in each scenario, whether optimistic or conservative flavor of the matrix; and unit costs for the three PWID interventions (NSP, MAT, and HCT). Since the costs of MAT overshadow the other unit costs, most of the total cost variation is due to this intervention. The standard deviation around the estimated cost in each country case was assumed for MAT to be US$100 around the mean. For impact matrix parameters, we modeled standard deviation of 40 percent around the point estimates shown in Tables 2.5 and 2.6.

For each of the three scenarios above, the uncertainty analysis is conducted by repeatedly sampling from a distribution constructed around the individual point value, and applying the sampled values in a run of the scenario in Goals.

We conduct at least 500 runs of each of the three scenarios to further describe the uncertainty in the modeled parameters. The median estimate and the 95 percent confidence intervals were computed for new infections and other reported results such as total costs, for each of the scenarios.

Cost-Effectiveness Analysis

Our intent was to inform decisions made by policymakers in countries to scale-up NSP, MAT, and HCT for PWID, as well as proportionate access to ART for PWID. In this context, we wanted to estimate the cost-effectiveness of increasing coverage of the interventions in an incremental manner, i.e., from a status quo to increasing access to ART, then further toward increased access and utilization of NSP, MAT, and HCT for PWID. The outcome of interest when comparing such scenarios is averted infection among PWID as well as at the community level. Using this outcome, we conducted an analysis to calculate the incremental cost-effectiveness ratio (ICER) in a stepped manner, comparing scenarios as they increase coverage incrementally.

Specifically, we compared the new infections under the status quo scenario to that under the baseline scenario and the "Expansion Optimistic" scenario; and then performed the same comparison for the baseline scenario and the "Expansion Conservative" and the "Expansion Optimistic" scenarios. The rationale for these comparisons is described in the context of each case study. Incremental cost-effectiveness ratios (ICER) were calculated as the scenarios change from the new infections averted and the added cost of increasing coverage from status quo to baseline, and from baseline to expansion. Uncertainty analysis was used to calculate the 95 percent confidence interval and the median value of these ICER results from 500 iterations of the model.

A Note on the Interpretation of ICER Values in the Context of Widely Used Thresholds: The use of thresholds related to GDP or GNI per capita are accepted for outcomes such as Quality-adjusted Life Years (QALY) or Disability-adjusted Life Years (DALY), following the Commission on the Macroeconomics of Health (WHO 2012). In the following case studies, we used these thresholds in the context of ICER related to an outcome of HIV infections averted. We note that HIV infections are closely related, in untreated HIV disease, to the risk of morbidity and mortality, both of which contribute to QALY and DALY calculations.

Data

Data availability for the countries being modeled was variable. We prioritized the use of national documents for target setting, where available, and relied on international documents such as the Universal Access targets and the WHO, UNODC, UNAIDS Technical Guide (WHO, UNODC et al. 2009) for countries to set targets for universal access to HIV prevention, treatment and care for injecting drug users. Data on risk behavior and population size were drawn from Demographic and Health Surveys, Behavioral Studies, and other country specific studies. These sources are cited in the individual case studies.

In most cases we were able to obtain baseline data to accurately represent coverage for the given services. In the remaining cases we used proxies from programs with a similar profile. Targets were aligned with National Strategic Plan for HIV/AIDS and program strategy documents.

Model Fitting

For HIV epidemic projections, we fit Goals to the official national projections, which were developed in Spectrum. The fitting process compared the HIV epidemic curves estimated within Goals to the curves from epidemic projections developed based on surveillance data and surveys. In other words, we would like to use Goals to simulate the epidemic curve (i.e., HIV prevalence over time) and compare it to the prevalence point estimates per year from a separate source. In order for us to trust its projection for future years, the model must be able to approximate, using mathematical modeling, the observed trend of the past years. We call this step "model fitting".

The prevalence point estimates by year are typically estimated by country teams working in collaboration with UNAIDS, using the Epidemic Projection Package now incorporated in the AIDS Impact Model within the Spectrum suite of models. The results of the fit are shown in each of the country case studies in the report.

Unit Costs

Country level unit costs were incorporated for interventions where available. Data from various sources were used for ART costs per patient year (see Appendix A for a list of sources), and a few inputs were derived from the Unit Cost Database (Futures Institute 2011). The unit costs of MAT and NSP per recipient per year were computed from available sources as well as derived from values used in recent studies (Schwartländer, Stover et al. 2011). In those cases where multiple data points were available from the Unit Cost Database, we used the one with the highest quality score.

Note

1. Since the time of this research, a global review of published and unpublished findings has been published, estimating an approximate 54% reduction in risk for HIV transmission associated with use of MAT (Macarthur et al. 2012). Given the timing of this publication and the research conducted for this report, the MacArthur estimates were not included in these modeling exercises; however, some of the same publications were also included in the estimated reduction in transmission of the impact matrix of Goals.

CHAPTER 3

Ukraine Case Study

Overview of the Epidemic

The first case of HIV in Ukraine was reported in 1987. There was rapid growth in the number of infected adults over the 1990s, and there was been much slower growth in the last decade. The country estimates that 181,609 HIV cases had been officially reported by January 2011 (0.57 percent of the 15–64 years old population). However, Ukraine's UNGASS 2010 report recognizes that the registry does not reflect the true size of the epidemic due to the number of Ukrainians who are unaware of their status or those who for some reason were not entered into the official national register of HIV infection cases (Ministry of Health Ukraine 2010). In fact, the UNGASS report suggests that the true estimate of all Ukrainians who were HIV-infected in 2010 is about 360,000 (1.1 percent of the 15–64 years old population, or 1.6 percent of the 15–49 years old population). Of this number, it is estimated that 77 percent are in the working-age population between 15 and 49 years old. The epidemic is unevenly distributed across the country, with a predominant proportion of the currently infected residing in the southeastern region, and thereafter in urban areas.

Ukraine's epidemic is at present a concentrated epidemic where there is less evidence of sustained transmission in the general, low-risk heterosexual population, but transmission continues to occur in certain key high-risk groups such as PWID, female sex workers (FSW), their clients, and men who have sex with men (MSM). In addition, there is secondary transmission to sexual partners of PWID as well as to the lower-risk regular partners of clients of commercial sex work. In this context, we believe that if transmission in these high-risk group groups is stabilized and then reversed, the levels of annual incidence will drop. There has been some success on this issue. A related change over time has been in the contribution of injecting drug use to incidence compared to sexual transmission.

Contribution of Injecting Drug Use to the Epidemic

There is some uncertainty over the number of Ukrainians who regularly inject drugs, whether opioids or non-opioids. Various estimates have been presented. The official, Ukrainian AIDS Center figures reported to the Reference Group to the United Nations on HIV and Injecting Drug Use (Mathers, Degenhardt et al. 2010) establish a low estimate of 0.71% of the population aged 15–64, to a high estimate of 1.12% on the same base. The mid-point estimate is 0.9%. This suggests a range from 227,670 to 359,140 drug injectors in Ukraine in 2011 using population numbers calculated in Spectrum's DemProj module. The population of PWID is heterogeneous. There is increasing diversity across type of drug, as well as age and gender.

There was sustained increase in opioid drug use during the 1990s, with an estimated peak in opioid use and initiation around 2000, based on surveys of students (15–16 year olds) as well as new presentations for drug dependence treatment (Vitek 2011). This pattern was mirrored by the estimated contribution of injecting drug use to HIV incidence which remained high till the mid-2000s. The UNGASS report and other sources suggest that the share of injecting drug use in overall transmission decreased from the mid-1990s. At some point in the mid-2000s, it fell below the share of sexual transmission. Modeling results vary on when this occurred; UNGASS report estimates that this occurred as late as 2009. Other studies suggest that the change had occurred earlier (Figure 3.1). The estimated year with the peak of HIV incidence specifically among PWID in terms of volume, was 1997 with approximately 7,500 infections (Ministry of Health Ukraine 2010).

The importance of modeling PWID and sexual transmission together cannot be overstated. The initial burst of infections among PWID in the 1990s was followed by a 'mirror wave' of infections among their sexual partners, mostly female (Vitek 2011).

As previously discussed, Goals allows for sexual risk among PWID to be modeled. In terms of their sexual risk behaviors, PWID are modeled as "medium risk", which allows for the averaging of some PWID with very high frequency of risky sexual behaviors, e.g., FSW who also inject, and others whose main risk behavior in the context of HIV is not sexual, but related to injecting drugs. Goals allows for overlapping of sexual and injecting risk behaviors through PWID and their sexual partners.

Figure 3.1   Estimated Relative Contribution of Sexual and PWID-Based Transmission to Overall Non-Vertical HIV Incidence (Left). Sources of Newly Registered HIV Cases, Including HIV-Exposed Infants (Mother-to-Child Transmission Or MTCT) (Right)

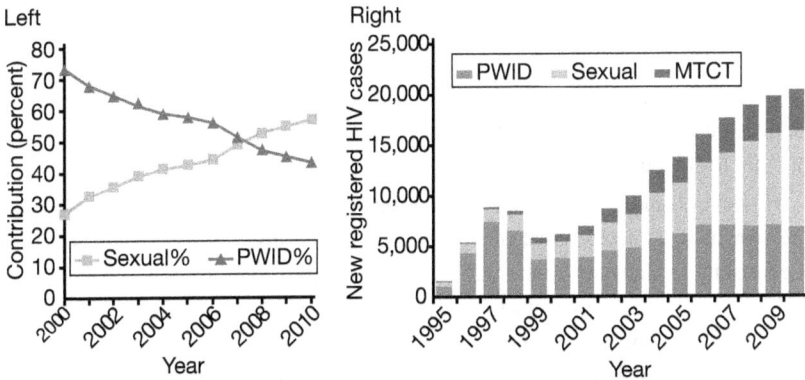

Sources: Left: Ministry of Health Ukraine 2010; Shulga 2011. Right: Vitek 2011.

Growing Heterogeneity in Injecting Drug Use in Ukraine

It is likely that the peak in opioid use and annual initiation in Ukraine occurred around 2000, and the trend has been the increasing importance of cocaine and stimulants in injecting drug use (Figure 3.2). A majority of PWID are male. Approximately 25 percent of all PWID are female. There is some indication that HIV prevalence among female PWID is higher than that among the male by a factor of approximately 1.4.

Figure 3.2   Primary Drug for Individuals Presenting for Treatment of Drug Addiction for the First Time

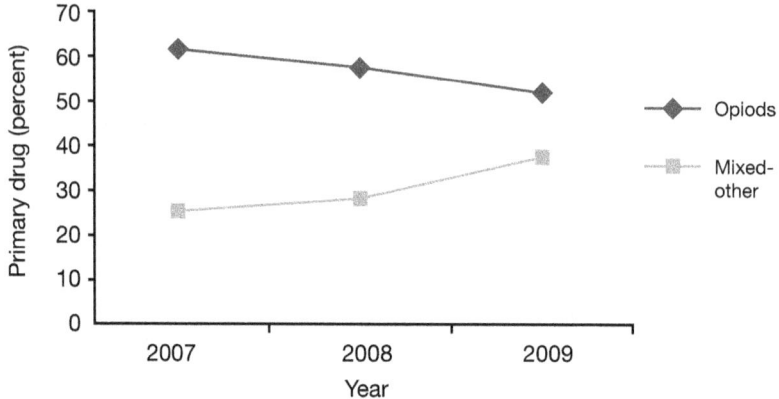

Source: Vitek 2011.

In surveys among students 15–16 years old, the percentage reporting ever using heroin or other opioids declined from a peak of 5.7 percent of the sample in 1999 to 0.5 percent in 2007. These facts are important for MAT scale-up.

However, opioid drugs still remain the primary injected substance due to the size of historical cohort of such injectors that continues in some form to the present. In a survey conducted by the Ukrainian chapter of the International HIV Alliance, 82 percent of PWID respondents reported injecting opioid extract or heroin, and 40 percent stimulants. There is overlap among the groups. Stimulants such as 'vint' (methamphetamine), 'jeff' (methcathinone), and 'boltushka' (cathinone) are used among younger PWID (Hurley 2010). The initial cohort of heroin and other opioid injectors has aged and there has been attrition from their ranks due to mortality and cessation of drug use. Therefore the PWID population today is more diverse than before, presenting challenges for HIV prevention policy.

Modeling Analysis

Model Fitting

Before estimating the effect of scaling up coverage for the four key interventions among PWID over 2012–2015, we required a model of the Ukrainian epidemic till 2011. This model fitting step was described in Chapter 2.

A 2012 version of the HIV epidemic curve fitted by the Ukraine country team working with UNAIDS, has not been released at the time of writing.

Such curves are estimated using seroprevalence surveillance data from key high-risk groups as well as antenatal clinic attendees incorporated in the Estimation and Projection Package (EPP). We compared the data on the national prevalence of HIV over time from previous UNAIDS reports, the country profile, and the most recent Ukraine UNGASS report to a curve fitted in Goals, which estimates annual national prevalence among the 15–49 year old population from behavioral risk and the size of different risk groups in the population, etc. The resulting curve is shown in Figure 3.3. This curve meets the expectations of a rapid rise in prevalence over the 1990s and a flattening of incidence and hence a slow rise in prevalence during the 2000s. It estimates a total of 319,580 HIV-positive adults between 15–49 years old in Ukraine in 2011, or 1.41 percent of the related population.

Figure 3.3   HIV-Positive Adults 15–49 Years Old in Ukraine From 1985–2011, as Modeled in Goals

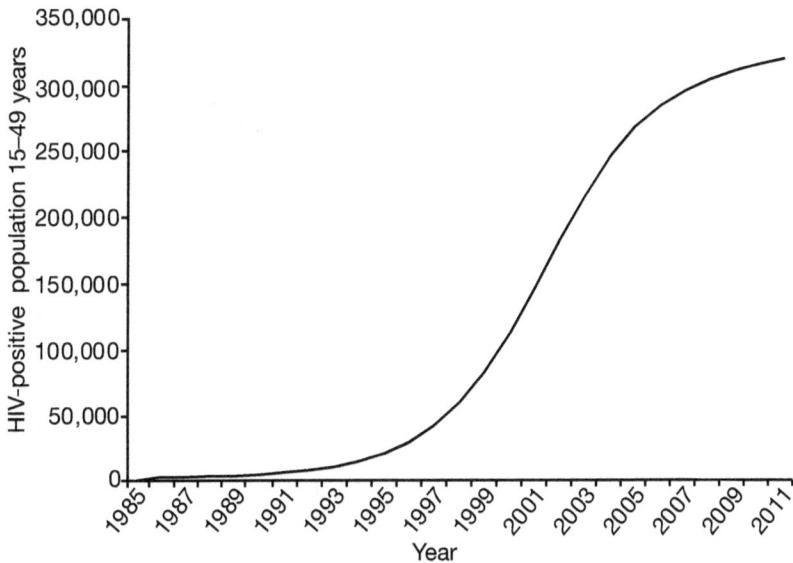

Source: Authors' calculations.

Population Size Estimates for PWID in Ukraine

As previously discussed, the UN Reference Group estimated range for the PWID population in Ukraine is 0.71 to 1.12 percent of the 15–64 age group with a mid-point estimate of 0.9 percent (IDU Reference Group 2010). However, Goals is a model that runs on the primary adult population of reproductive and working age, i.e., 15–49 years. As previously stated, it takes as inputs fixed percentages of the adult population that fall in various risk groups, by gender. These percentages are applied to the estimated male and female adult population, per year. In order to satisfy this input requirement, we calculated the proportion of the PWID group that fell in the 15–49 age group starting from the beginning of the HIV epidemic in 1985. We assumed that the average age of the PWID population has increased over time, commensurate with anecdotal accounts of aging in the original opioid-injecting groups, which implies a declining proportion in the age group 15–49.

While the UN Reference Group estimates based on official figures are not gender-disaggregated percentages, Goals requires separate percentage estimates for male and female PWID. Based on available information, we assumed that the PWID population has become increasingly male, even from historically high levels. These assumptions result in estimated sizes of male and female PWID population 15–49 years in Goals per year. These values were used as the denominators for determining coverage levels for interventions.

Figure 3.4   PWID Population Estimates in Ukraine from Goals Modeling (Adult PWID 15–49 Years Old) and UN Reference Group Range/Midpoint (All PWID 15–64 Years Old)

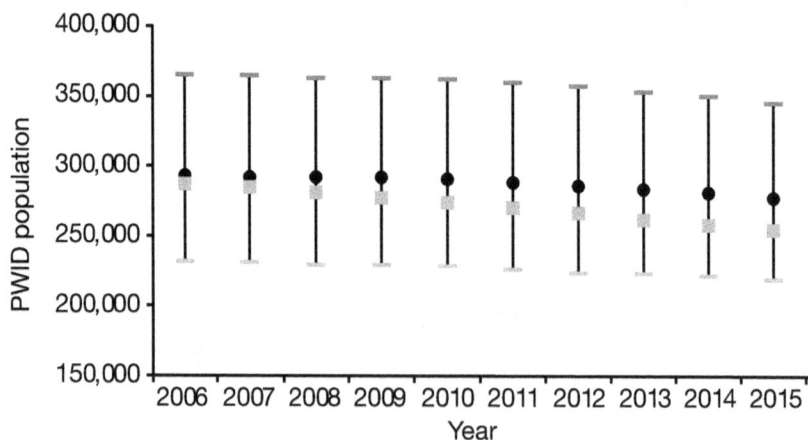

Source: Authors' calculations, IDU Reference Group 2010.

Figure 3.4 compares the total population size (summing male and female PWID) from Goals to the UN Reference Group range and midpoint estimate and shows the range of values for PWID population size in Ukraine. It shows our PWID size estimate from Goals, utilizing the demographic projection of adult population 15–49 year old per year and the fixed percentage estimate of the proportion of PWID in the population, disaggregated by gender. We expected that the UN Reference Group estimate would be larger, as it covers the 15–64 year range for PWID and the gap between the midpoint estimate and the Goals estimate increases over time, as we would expect from the increasing aging of the PWID population.

Scenarios

Modeling scenarios were described in Chapter 2. We modeled the Status Quo, Baseline, and the two versions of the Expansion scenario. It is important to distinguish the Baseline and the Expansion scenarios in terms of the coverage for NSP, MAT, HCT, and ART interventions.

The Status Quo scenario maintains ART, NSP, MAT, and HCT coverage at the levels seen in 2011 (i.e., 25,120). Only ART coverage increases in the Baseline scenario. Coverage levels are described in Table 3.1 below. In the Baseline scenario, coverage for all key PWID interventions is expected to remain stable over 2011–2015, except for adult ART, where a scale-up path has already been listed by the government and partners using Global Fund and other resources. In the Baseline scenario, it is assumed that PWID now achieve a proportionate share in ART coverage, as described in Chapter 2.

Table 3.1   Status Quo and Baseline Scenarios for Key Interventions among PWID in Ukraine

Intervention	2011	2012	2013	2014	2015
ART: status quo	25,120				
ART: baseline	25,120	25,284	29,268	33,252	37,235
HCT for PWID[b]	40.5 % of PWID (Ministry of Health Ukraine 2010)				
NSP[b]	52 % of all PWID (Ministry of Health Ukraine 2010)				
MAT[b]	2.6 %[a] of all opioid-dependent PWID (Ministry of Health Ukraine 2010; HIV/AIDS 2011; Vitek 2011)				

Source: Authors.
Note: ART = antiretroviral therapy; HCT = HIV counseling and testing; MAT = medically assisted therapy; NSP = needle and syringe program.
a. Authors' calculations in goals of PWID population, and applying opioid-using proportion of 89 percent.
b. Same across status quo and baseline scenarios.

As of September 2011, there were 6,390 PWID on MAT in Ukraine—12 percent on BMT and 88 percent on MMT. Of these, 881 individuals also received ART, or 14 percent of the total on MAT. In 2008, a total of 132,361 people were reached by NSP distributing sterile needles or syringes, approximately 47 percent of all PWID, using the population size estimate from Goals as a denominator. In 2010, the stated program coverage for "sterile needles/syringes plus condoms received in the last 12 months" among PWID was 52 percent. All of these data are from official Ukrainian sources.

In the Baseline scenario, coverage levels for HCT, NSP, and MAT are maintained over 2012–2015 as in the table above. The Goals model was run for the Status Quo and Baseline scenarios and uncertainty analysis was conducted.

Table 2.1 in Chapter 2 described the scale-up ranges proposed in the WHO/UNODC/UNAIDS 'technical guide' (WHO, UNODC et al. 2009). We set a scale-up path from 2012–2015 for Ukraine for the four key interventions. The choice of the final endpoint in 2015 for coverage was based on an estimate of what was the appropriate target given current coverage, and what was needed.

For NSP, we set the target as 75 percent coverage of all PWID, which is in the "High" range from the guide. We assumed a linear expansion path from current 2011 coverage to this value over the four years 2012–2015. For MAT, given the low coverage currently, we set a scale-up target of 15 percent by 2015, drawing from the "Low" range of the technical guide. We programmed a linear scale-up path to this target from the current level of 2.6 percent of all opioid-injecting individuals. For HCT, we set a target of 60 percent of PWID from the "Medium" range. The results are listed in Table 3.2 for the Expansion scenarios.

Table 3.2   Expansion Scenario Coverage for the Four Key Interventions among PWID in Ukraine

Intervention	2011	2012	2013	2014	2015
ART	25,120	25,284	29,268	33,252	37,235
HCT for PWID	41%	48%	52%	56%	60%
NSP	52%	58%	64%	70%	75%
MAT	2.6%	6.4%	8.5%	11%	15%

Source: Authors.
Note: ART = antiretroviral therapy; HCT = HIV counseling and testing; MAT = medically assisted therapy; NSP = needle and syringe program.

Results

Extending the epidemic curve shown in Figure 3.3 would reflect a slowing in the rate of growth of new HIV infections in Ukraine due to a variety of reasons. These include the shrinking size of the PWID population, continuing improvements in prevention among heterosexual couples, as well as the recent trend of antiretroviral treatment scale-up. In this context, total new HIV infections among adult male and female PWID will increase slowly after 2011. Ideally, these values should decline. We find that with the expansion in the coverage of the four key PWID interventions—ART, HCT for PWID, NSP, and MAT—new HIV infections among PWID do decline further (Figure 3.5).

Figure 3.5   New HIV Infections among PWID in Ukraine—Comparison across Modeled Scenarios

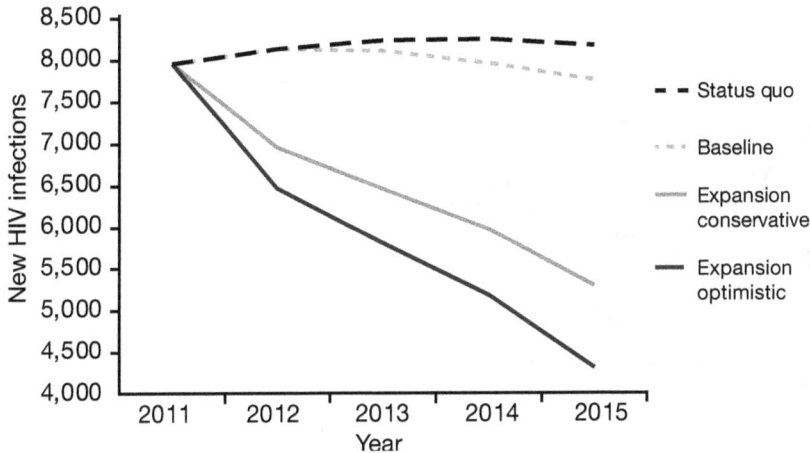

Source: Authors' calculations.

Figure 3.5 reveals considerable effects in terms of averted HIV infections among PWID from the expansion of NSP, MAT, and HCT for PWID, along with the equitable provision of ART to PWID. While the figure is concerned with infections among PWID, there are also moderate reductions in community infections via effects in the overlapping sexual and injecting networks. Table 11 demonstrates this with the compiled results for averted adult (15–49 years) HIV infections, comparing different pairs of scenarios.

Table 3.3   Averted HIV Infections Among Adults 15–49 Years Old in Ukraine, by Modeled Scenario

Year	Compared to status quo		Compared to baseline	
	Baseline	Expansion optimistic	Expansion conservative	Expansion optimistic
2012	25	1,728	1,199	1,703
2013	630	3,086	1,759	2,456
2014	1,356	4,426	2,202	3,070
2015	2,007	5,910	2,797	3,903
Overall	4,018	15,150	7,957	11,132

Source: Authors.

Over 2012–2015, the Expansion scenario, regardless of the impact matrix variety, costs approximately an additional US$75 million over the Baseline scenario. The Baseline scenario costs an additional US$2.5 million over the Status Quo scenario. Given these additional costs, we can now conduct cost-effectiveness analysis. Table 3.4 provides the incremental cost-effectiveness ratios (ICER) for the same comparisons as performed in Table 3.3.

Table 3.4   Incremental Cost-Effectiveness Ratios, US$ per Averted Adult Infection, Ukraine

Year	Compared to status quo		Compared to baseline	
	Baseline	Expansion optimistic	Expansion conservative	Expansion optimistic
2012	$4,445	$5,705	$8,129	$5,723
2013	$999	$4,984	$8,396	$6,006
2014	$997	$4,950	$9,357	$6,697
2015	$155	$5,110	$10,100	$7,658
Overall	$598	$5,105	$9,221	$6,732

Source: Authors.

In the language of cost-effectiveness analysis, Baseline dominates the Expansion Optimistic scenario when the base of comparisons to Status Quo. Offering equitable access to PWID in ART is extremely cost-effective, with an ICER less than Ukraine's Gross National Income (GNI) per capita at purchasing power parity of US$6,580 (World Bank 2010). This applies the WHO-CHOICE threshold (WHO 2012).

We need to interpret the value of expanding NSP, MAT, and HCT for PWID when this is incremental to offering proportionate access for PWID to ART. Table 3.4 suggests that such additional scale-up, adding to a combination prevention approach for PWID, is cost-effective. Expansion Optimistic dominates the Expansion Conservative scenario, when the base for averted infections and incremental costs is the Baseline scenario. The ICER for both Expansion Scenarios in comparisons to the Baseline scenario is less than three times the GNI per capita. Overall, if the effectiveness of the three interventions in reducing risky behavior among PWID approaches levels seen in developed countries, then expansion in their coverage is quite cost-effective (US$6,732 from Table 10 is close to the GNI per capita).

Uncertainty Analysis

We ran 500 iterations for each scenario, varying the impact matrix parameters and unit costs, resulting in distributions for various model outputs. We recorded the medians and the 95 percent confidence intervals (CI) for new HIV infections and total costs for each scenario. Comparing scenarios, we created Figure 3.6.

Figure 3.6   Overall ICER for Ukraine Scenarios 2012–15: Median, 95 Percent CI

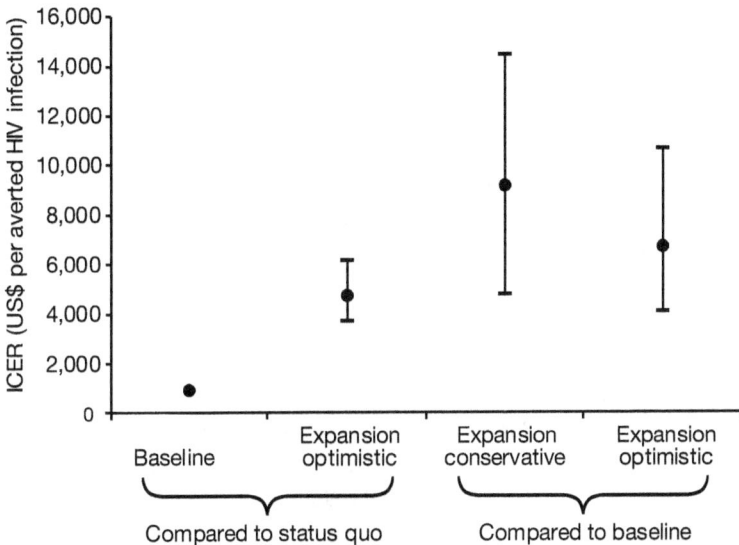

Source: Authors.
Note: ICER = incremental cost-effectiveness ratio.

We interpreted the results of the uncertainty analysis in light of the values in Table 3.4. We have a good degree of confidence that the ICER for the Baseline scenario compared to Status Quo (no scale-up) shows that providing equitable access to PWID in ART scale-up is extremely cost-effective. We are also confident that Expansion of NSP, MAT, and HCT for PWID in comparison to flat coverage under the Baseline scenario is cost-effective (i.e., below a double multiple of the GNI per capita from Ukraine). These conclusions are further strengthened if we believe that Ukrainian implementers can reach levels of effectiveness in their programs for NSP, MAT, and HCT for PWID comparable to those seen in the West.

Discussion

Ukraine has made strong progress in scaling up programs providing outreach services, including interventions to provide sterile needles, syringes and other injecting equipment to PWID. Further progress is needed, especially in raising the coverage of MAT from its currently low levels. Our results show that such scale-up is cost-effective even at moderate levels of intervention impact, and very cost-effective at higher levels of effectiveness. This study corroborates finding from other modeling studies for Ukraine which adopted a different methodology and found the scale-up of MAT alongside ART at very high levels to be very cost-effective in Ukraine (Alistar, Owens et al. 2011).

Our model shows that if Ukraine increases coverage for NSP to 75 percent and HCT for PWID to 60 percent, with proportionate provision of ART to PWID and 15 percent coverage of MAT among opiate-dependent PWID, then it can reduce new infections in this group by 34 percent compared to status quo at 2011 levels of coverage. This depends on the interventions being highly effective—a requirement that Ukrainian implementers can meet, but not without some change to the overall policy environment. This reduction is in the range established for Ukrainian cities by other studies modeling similar scale-up of NSP, MAT, and equitable access to ART (Strathdee, Hallett et al. 2010).

While we do not model structural factors, other studies have done so (Strathdee, Hallett et al. 2010), and they suggest that removal of punitive provisions against PWID in Ukrainian cities such as Odessa can ameliorate the risk environment, diminish stigma, and reduce the risk of HIV acquisition. Besides such benefits in epidemic control, reducing problematic police practices related to PWID is an important human rights issue.

CHAPTER 4

Pakistan Case Study

Overview of the Epidemic

Pakistan has a concentrated HIV epidemic, and sustained transmission has been occurring in specific high-risk groups since the 1990s. These groups have been tracked through successive seroprevalence and behavioral studies in different cities, as a result of which there is a good body of evidence. The high-risk groups, sometimes referred to as "core" groups, were initially identified through such surveys and local epidemiological studies. They are female sex workers (FSW), male sex workers (MSW), *hijra* or transgender sex workers (HSW), and PWID. In addition to these four groups, there are a few other groups at a risk of HIV higher than the general population: truck drivers and allied transport workers, and migrants inclusive of refugees.

There is evidence that the transmission of HIV in the general low-risk population is limited. There have been clusters of infections due to infected blood and blood products, but the continuing importance of this channel in incidence may be limited. The national second generation surveillance (SGS) activity in 2011 conducted a seroprevalence survey in antenatal clinics with a sample size of 27,000 women. The result indicated an antenatal HIV prevalence of 0.05 percent, which is line with previous estimates for the low-risk adult population in Pakistan (Dar 2012). Risk is considered to be higher than the general population among certain 'bridging' populations, though evidence in terms of HIV seroprevalence surveys is limited. These bridging groups have been defined as truck drivers, clients of FSW, and migrants (Khan and Khan 2010). The two provinces of Punjab and Sindh, which account for 81 percent of Pakistan's population as well as the largest urban centers, also have most of the high-risk groups.

Given the nature of the epidemic and the history of its evolution, prevention strategy focused heavily on the four high-risk groups. The Government of Pakistan began the Enhanced HIV/AIDS Control Program (EHACP-1) with own and development partner funding in 2003. This continued till 2008. A break in key outreach and prevention programs mostly implemented by NGO occurred in 2009, with the end of the key development partner financing mechanism. More recently, the prevention program management has deconcentrated to a provincial level. The "PC1" mechanism allocates federal funds to provinces for approved development projects, and has been funding limited HIV programs since 2008 for the four high-risk groups as well as limited treatment and care interventions. These were supplemented by funds from the GFATM Round 2 grant. The recent GFATM Round 9 grant is expected to increase coverage of interventions, with additional services funded by the PC-1 mechanism. However, substantial gaps in coverage are still expected to occur, as discussed later.

Contribution of Injecting Drug Use to the Epidemic

Formal modes of transmission analyses have not been undertaken for Pakistan, but a recent scenario modeling study estimated that PWID could contribute between 15 to 32 percent of HIV incidence by 2015 in Karachi, and 15 to 30 percent of incidence in Lahore, depending on assumptions (Emmanuel 2012). This mirrors a fact widely acknowledged that PWID contribute a significant proportion of new infections in the country. Most of the prevention resources in the country over 2008–2009 were spent on programs for PWID (NACP 2010b). Drug use has increased following increasing inflows of opiates from Afghanistan from the 1990s. More of the drug users began to inject rather than smoking or inhaling opiates, which is a function both of increasing dependency as well as shifts in preferences (Nai Zindagi 2008). Most PWID in Pakistan are street-based, and group injecting practices are common, with expert users ("street doctors") injecting many. Recent SGS suggests that as many as 70 percent of all PWID were injected by a street doctor in the month prior to survey (Emmanuel and Reza 2012).

There are well-documented reports of risk behaviors such as sharing of injecting equipment and large sharing groups. Behavioral surveillance in a sample of Pakistani cities indicated that rates of sharing—a critical risk behavior—were very high historically but declined in the period when interventions scaled up (Figure 10). In the period 2004–2008, ecological studies indicate that NGO-driven outreach and NSP programs for PWID were effective in reducing such risk behavior and had a peak coverage in terms of PWID registered of 26 percent across five provinces (Khan and Khan 2011). However, coverage in terms of the needle and syringe need was highly variable across the targeted cities, and the interventions were also expensive. The HIV prevalence among PWID in the cities did not decline during the period of the interventions, which mostly ended in 2009 with the cessation of external funding.

Figure 4.1   Estimated National Proportion of PWID Sharing Needles/Syringes from SGS Rounds

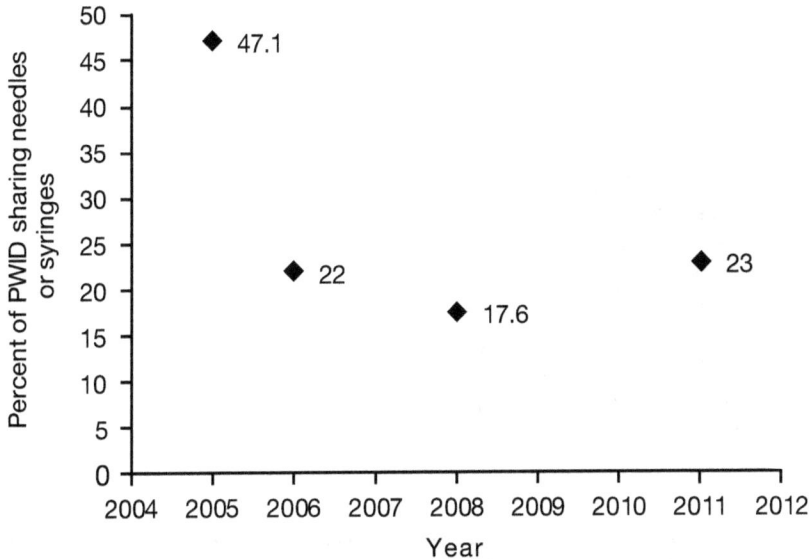

Sources: NACP 2005; NACP 2007; NACP 2008; Emmanuel and Reza 2012.
Note: SGS = second generation surveillance.

A study of the experience with the NSP and outreach response led by NGO over 2005– 2007 suggests several factors that could have contributed to a lack of reduction in HIV prevalence. These include the short duration of the interventions, the movement of PWID between cities with differing intervention coverage, and problems in targeting of the interventions towards all age brackets of PWID (Khan and Khan 2011). The study also comments on the design of the average NSP intervention during this period, where a lack of resources may have meant inadequate supplementation of needle/syringe supply with counseling. The lack of an integrated, combination approach, without available voluntary HCT, also suggests a lack of effect on key HIV prevention outcomes.

In recent years, the spread of HIV among PWID has been recorded in the form of growing or emerging epidemics in non-traditional areas such as medium-sized urban centers in four provinces and districts in provinces other than Punjab or Sindh (Pakistan Harm Reduction Technical Advisory Committee 2012).

Population Size Estimates for PWID in Pakistan

The UN Reference Group estimated that Pakistan had 135,000 PWID (range 141,000–162,500) in 2008, which equated to 0.14 percent of the population 15–64 years (IDU Reference Group 2010). As previously stated, the Goals model concerns the adult working and reproductive age population aged 15–49 years. We assume a population size of 112,500 PWID aged 15–49 years, predominantly male (98 percent). The gender split was informed by the latest SGS round (Emmanuel and Reza 2012).This corresponded to 0.23 percent of the 15–49 year old male population in 2010, and 0.005 percent of the similar female population.

Table 4.1   Different Population Size Estimates for PWID in Pakistan

Estimate	Source	Year of estimate
80,000–145,000	Khan and Khan 2010	2010
141,000–162,500	IDU Reference Group 2010	2008
91,000	NACP 2010b	2006–2007
112,500[a]	Current study	2011
39,793–52,896[b]	Emmanuel 2012	2011 (not national)

Source: Authors; see Source column.
Note: IDU = injecting drug user; NACP = National AIDS Control Programme.
a. National estimate, for age group 15–49 years.
b. Estimate for 19 cities in Pakistan only

Based on the SGS Round 4 (2011), we assumed approximately 46 percent of male PWID were married. Transmission of HIV to spouses of PWID is a concern, and this parameter allows for this channel to be modeled. We also assumed that about 60 percent of PWID in Pakistan inject opiates, based on SGS Round 3 (NACP 2008). Poly drug use is common among Pakistani PWID. A variety of opiates such as heroin and drugs such as tamgesic, bupron, and sosegon are injected as well as anti-histamines and narcotic analgesics. Popularity of different drugs differs by region, and opiate use can be high or low.

Modeling Analysis

Model Fitting

As the recent SGS Round 4 suggests, HIV in Pakistan continues to be driven by PWID, among whom HIV has "established a firm foothold" and has recently intensified; as well as MSW and HSW, among which the epidemic is expanding quickly" (Emmanuel 2012). For successive historical SGS rounds, HIV prevalence among FSW remained low, but there is some indication of an increasing trend based on the rise in the statistic from 0.4 percent to 0.8 percent between SGS Round 1 and Round 4.

We collected data on sexual behavior—condom use, number of partners per year, and number of sex acts per partner—for FSW, MSW, HSW, and lower-risk groups. These parameters were discussed in Chapter 2. The data for both HSW and MSW from SGS rounds were combined in weighted averages for most of the sexual parameters, since we used a single MSM-related risk group in the model. Weights were the group sizes per year. In addition, we used available data on sexually transmitted infections for all the risk groups in the model. As discussed previously for Ukraine (Chapter 3), PWID are modeled as "medium risk" for their sexual behavior. In the case of Pakistan, this is supported by the recent SGS. Nearly 14 percent of PWID reported contact with FSW in the six months prior to the survey, and reported condom use was low (17 percent).

We compare the prevalence curves for key high-risk groups to the recent national estimates from SGS rounds (Figure 4.2). In addition, we compared the modeled national adult epidemic curve from Goals to a curve fitted in a recent exercise using the Spectrum AIDS Epidemic Model (Figure 4.3).

Figure 4.2   Comparison of Model and Survey-Based HIV Prevalence Estimates in Pakistan From 2001–11 for PWID (Left) and for MSW/HSW (Weighted Average) (Right)

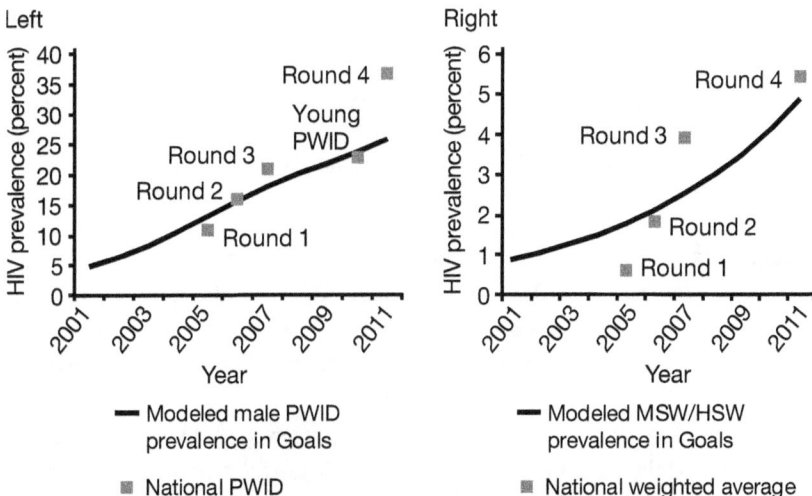

Sources: Authors' calculations; NACP 2005; NACP 2007; NACP 2008; NACP 2010a; Emmanuel and Reza 2012.
Note: HSW = hijra sex worker; MSW = male sex worker.

Our model is conservative in terms of the estimated HIV prevalence for PWID in recent years. We avoided over-fitting the model to the recent spike in PWID prevalence seen in SGS Round 4, as it caused the national prevalence estimate to be overestimated. The national epidemic curve is shown in Figure 4.3.

Figure 4.3   HIV-Positive Adults 15–49 Years Old in Pakistan From 1985–2011, as Modeled in Goals

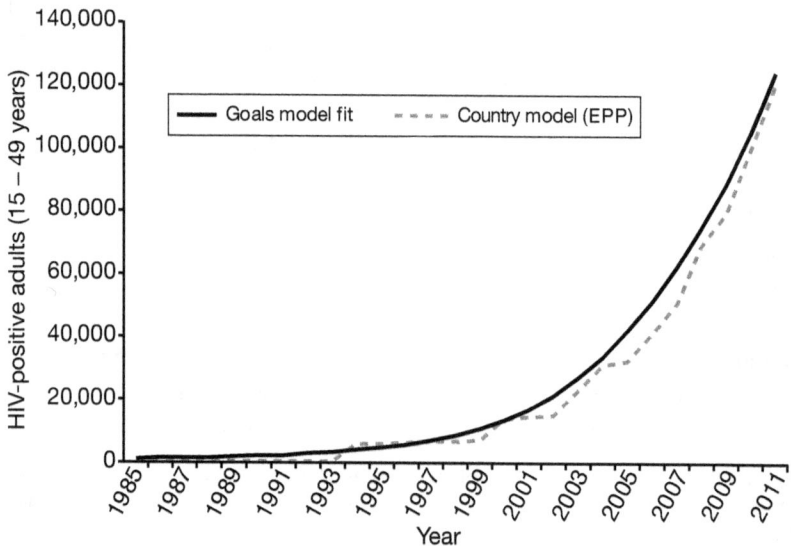

Source: Authors' calculations, Pakistan country team/UNAIDS.
Note: EPP = estimation and projection package.

Our model estimates national HIV prevalence among adults in Pakistan 15–49 years old to be 0.13 percent, equivalent to 0.11 percent of the 15–64 years old population. This is close to the official estimate.

Scenarios

Modeling scenarios were described in Chapter 2. We modeled the Status Quo, Baseline, and the two versions of the Expansion scenario. It is important to distinguish the Baseline and the Expansion scenarios in terms of the coverage for NSP, MAT, HCT, and ART interventions.

The GFATM Round 2 grant enabled Pakistan to start 13 ART centers in tertiary hospitals and 16 HCT sites. The last UNGASS report put the number of PLWHA being provided free ART in 2009 at 1,320 (NACP 2010b). Per the scale-up plan currently filed with UNAIDS, the number of individuals on ART in 2011 had increased to 2,015. Table 4.2 describes the Status Quo and Baseline scenarios. For the former, ART coverage is fixed at the value from 2011. In the Baseline scenario, this increases, per the established scale-up plan.

There is little evidence to suggest that prior to 2011 any significant fraction of HIV-positive and eligible PWID had access to HIV care and treatment. In the Baseline scenario, as previously discussed, it is assumed PWID now have equi-proportionate access to the intervention as it scales up. The coverage levels for NSP, MAT, and HCT for PWID related to the start year (2011) were estimated based on the scale achieved in the PC-1 programs as well as the planned start-up of activities under the GFATM Round 9 grant. This scale was maintained over the course of 2012–2015 for these two scenarios.

Table 4.2   Status Quo and Baseline Scenarios for Key Interventions among PWID in Pakistan

Intervention	2011	2012	2013	2014	2015
ART: status quo	2,015				
ART: baseline	2,015	2,400	2,785	3,170	3,555
HCT for PWID[a]	17% of PWID				
NSP[a]	18% of PWID				
MAT[a]	Not provided (zero coverage)				

Source: Authors.
Note: ART = antiretroviral therapy; HCT = HIV counseling and testing; MAT = medically assisted therapy; NSP = needle and syringe program.
a. Same across status quo and baseline scenarios. Values based on estimated size of PWID population in 2011.

There was some delay in the start of the GFATM Round 9 grant, and in the period 2010–2011, the contract providing for certain PWID interventions in the Punjab province under the previous national strategy also came to an end. Therefore, program coverage in 2011 begins from a low base. Some scale-up in the interventions is expected under GFATM Round 9 implementation, with additional coverage being provided under the PC-1 mechanism. We calculated the total coverage under these plans as a percentage of the estimated national PWID population per year from Goals.

The GFATM Round 9 grant was awarded separately to two Principal Recipients: the Nai Zindagi Trust, a NGO from Lahore, and the National AIDS Control Program (NACP). Under its grant, Nai Zindagi has committed to a scale-up of NSP to reach 17,900 PWID by the end of March 2013 (GFATM 2011). The NACP grant covers ART for PWID and other treatment and care services for PLWHA. Nai Zindagi primarily services PWID in Punjab, which means that gaps exist for NSP in other provinces. The total coverage from

GFATM and PC-1 sources for NSP in 2012 is planned to be in the range of 28,500 (11,500 and 17,000 respectively). These figures are based on recent proposals (CCM Pakistan 2009). The value 28,500 corresponds to coverage of 25 percent nationally. Even with these generous estimates, we calculate that coverage for NSP will only be 37 percent nationally by 2015, much of it uncertain.

The GFATM Round 9 grant, along with PC-1, intends to offer a comprehensive "service delivery package" to PWID, which includes MAT. Pakistan intends to begin a pilot MAT program from 2013 at one or two selected sites. During 2012, initial scoping exercises would be conducted and necessary clearances obtained to use buprenorphine. Based on available data and our calculation, the scale of coverage was expected to reach only 3 percent of opiate-injecting PWID in Pakistan nationally by 2015.

We programmed a more ambitious scale-up plan that would reach 60 percent coverage for NSP and HCT for PWID by 2015, drawing the value from the "Medium" range of the Technical Guide (WHO, UNODC et al. 2009). For MAT, we targeted 20 percent coverage among PWID ("Low" range), adjusting for the proportion of opiate-injecting individuals. Annual targets were estimated based on a linear scale-up path from 2012 to 2015. Results are used for Expansion scenarios in our modeling and are shown in Table 4.3.

Table 4.3   Expansion Scenario Coverage for the Four Key Interventions among PWID in Pakistan

Intervention	2011	2012	2013	2014	2015
ART	2,015	2,400	2,785	3,170	3,555
HCT for PWID	17%	28%	38%	49%	60%
NSP	18%	28%	39%	49%	60%
MAT	0%	5%	10%	15%	20%

Source: Authors.
Note: ART = antiretroviral therapy; HCT = HIV counseling and testing; MAT = medically assisted therapy; NSP = needle and syringe program.

Results

The epidemic curve in Figure 4.3 shows an increasing HIV prevalence level among adults nationally, driven by continuing transmission in the four key high-risk groups, and especially due to recent trends among PWID following the interruption in harm reduction services. The scale-up planned under GFATM Round 9 and the PC-1 mechanism will help to slow incidence over

2012–2015, but more can and should be done, as Pakistani experts suggested (Pakistan Harm Reduction Technical Advisory Committee 2012).

Comparing Status Quo to the Baseline scenario, the availability of proportionate access for PWID in ART scale-up has little effect on infections in the group due to the small scale of the ART intervention overall. In our model, the coverage among PWID eligible for ART at the current threshold in Pakistan of CD4 t-cells below 350 cells per mm^3 rises from between 4 and 5 percent in the Status Quo scenario to 6 percent in the Baseline scenario. This also reflects the modeling of other PLWHA eligible for ART, from non-PWID risk groups, getting their share of the intervention.

The rise in coverage for ART among PWID is insufficient to create major change in the incidence in the group. Pakistan needs to scale up ART further. However, we find that with the expansion in the coverage of three of the four key PWID interventions—HCT for PWID, NSP, and MAT—new HIV infections among PWID decline sharply (Figure 4.4).

Figure 4.4   New HIV Infections among PWID in Pakistan—Comparison across Modeled Scenarios

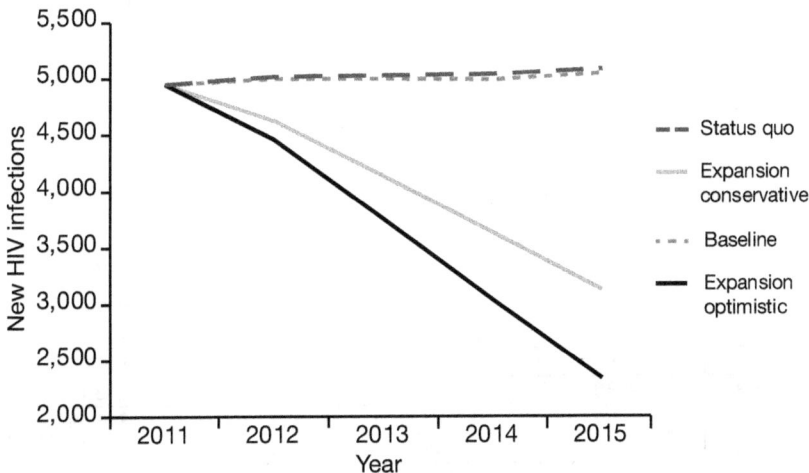

Source: Authors' calculations.

While Figure 4.4 suggests ART scale-up alone is not effective for reduction in incidence among PWID at the current scale, it does lead to modest reductions in incidence more broadly across all risk groups in Goals, as shown in Table 4.4 (Baseline compared to Status Quo). In 2015, Pakistan's current

ART scale-up program averts 556 HIV infections among adults compared to a situation where ART coverage is held at 2011 levels. Table 4.5 shows the overall compiled results by year for averted adult HIV infections.

Table 4.4   Averted HIV Infections among Adults 15–49 Years Old in Pakistan, by Modeled Scenario

Year	Compared to status quo		Compared to baseline	
	Baseline	Expansion optimistic	Expansion conservative	Expansion optimistic
2012	93	429	166	336
2013	233	906	258	673
2014	379	1,572	502	1,193
2015	556	4,686	3,152	4,130
Overall	1,261	7,593	4,078	6,332

Source: Authors.

Over 2012–2015, the Expansion scenario, regardless of the impact matrix variety, costs approximately an additional US$62 million over the Baseline scenario. The Baseline scenario costs approximately another US$1 million compared to the Status Quo scenario. Given these additional costs, we conduct cost-effectiveness analysis. Table 4.5 below provides the ICER for the same comparisons as in Table 4.4.

Table 4.5   Incremental Cost-Effectiveness Ratios, US$ per Averted Adult Infection, Pakistan

Year	Compared to status quo		Compared to baseline	
	Baseline	Expansion optimistic	Expansion conservative	Expansion optimistic
2012	$382	$15,786	$40,582	$20,050
2013	$580	$14,071	$48,902	$18,743
2014	$555	$11,968	$37,080	$15,594
2015	$495	$5,266	$7,749	$5,908
Overall	$520	$8,299	$15,300	$9,848

Source: Authors.

Baseline dominates the Expansion Optimistic scenario when the base scenario is Status Quo. This is mostly due to averted infections in non-PWID groups and based on the small incremental cost of scaling up ART to low levels of coverage. Expansion Optimistic averts more infections at a higher total cost. Compared to a Status Quo, scaling up ART is very cost-effective but does little for PWID infections at current scale of provision. Adding scale-up of NSP, MAT, and HCT (Expansion Optimistic) is cost-effective compared to Status Quo, given Pakistan's GNI per capita at purchasing power parity of US$2,800 (World Bank 2010). However, high effectiveness may be difficult to achieve from the start.

Should Pakistan add scale-up of NSP, MAT, and HCT for PWID over and above the scale-up in adult ART? Since we are interested in combination prevention for PWID, accessing the other three key interventions from a harm reduction services package is essential. In this context, when the comparison is to the Baseline scenario, Expansion Optimistic dominates the Expansion Conservative scenario. The former scenario averts 4,130 infections among adults 15–49 years in 2015 compared to Baseline. But, the two scenarios overall across 2012–2015 are not cost-effective as per the WHO-CHOICE threshold.

The individual ICER values for 2015 ($7,749 and $5,908 respectively for the two Expansion scenarios) suggest that such additions to the combination prevention package can become cost-effective over time. The unit costs we have used build in initial higher costs to cater to program setup (see Appendix A). Economies of scale and other efficiencies come later. Pakistan should attempt to reduce initial costs of start-up to make the expansion in combination prevention for PWID even more cost-effective.

Uncertainty Analysis

Are the interpretations above susceptible to uncertainty in model parameters, especially unit costs? We conducted the uncertainty analysis as in the Ukraine case study (Chapter 3). Figure 4.5 shows the results. The figure suggests that conclusions above should stand and are not affected by parametric uncertainty.

Figure 4.5   Overall ICER for Pakistan Scenarios 2012–15: Median, 95 Percent CI

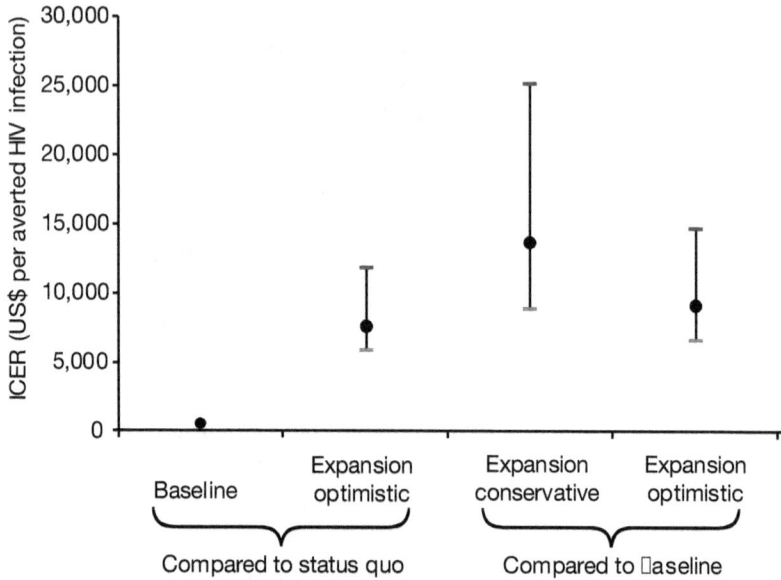

Source: Authors.
Note: ICER = incremental cost-effectiveness ratio.

Discussion

Following the reduction in external funding from 2009, the recent history till 2011 for harm reduction interventions in Pakistan has been one of intermittent starts and stops. In May 2010, EHACP-1 contractual agreements in Punjab province broke down and NSP and outreach services went from a planned extension to eight cities (with a potential for an additional four cities) to isolated, small programs funded by UNODC and other donors, covering around 1,000 PWID.

A similar scenario befell Sindh province, where EHACP-1 coverage of NSP and outreach interventions ended at the close of 2009. The Government of Pakistan assumed funding for certain PWID services in Karachi, the biggest city in Sindh, until the end of 2010. Thereafter in Karachi the NGOs Pakistan Society and Al-Nijat continued limited services through their own resources until early 2011. Again, UNAIDS and UNODC provided bridge funding to enable coverage of NSP and outreach programs for about 7,000 PWID till PC-1 based mechanisms could take over funding. Another 1,000 PWID were reached by Interact World Wide. Such coverage levels are simply too small given a low estimate of 44,000 PWID in the major cities of Punjab and Sindh alone (Emmanuel and Reza 2012).

Data from these two largest provinces are scarce to establish the design, effectiveness, and costs of harm reduction services offered and utilized in the period 2009–2011. For example, there is little knowledge whether coverage was effective in terms of needles and syringes supplied compared to the need. In our modeling of coverage, we assumed a low base to begin the scale-up from 2012. In this context, the GFATM Round 9 grant presents a major opportunity to increase high-quality coverage for the key harm reduction interventions: NSP, HCT for PWID, as well as ART. Eventually, MAT will also be provided, though at small scale. The Principal Recipients—Nai Zindagi Trust and the NACP—have begun project implementation in certain districts of Punjab and Sindh from the first quarter of 2012.

However, even with these scale-up plans, primarily funded with external resources, the overall coverage of these four key interventions for PWID is too low and poorly distributed. Emerging centers of HIV infection among PWID in Pakistan are not being addressed. Pakistani stakeholders have done a good job of defining a comprehensive service delivery package for PWID, addressing the HIV risk as well as the broad health outcomes of this group. It is now time to implement it at scale and curb the likelihood of continuing rise in the number of HIV infections in the country.

With NSP and HCT for PWID at 60 percent coverage by 2015, proportionate access for PWID in ART scale-up, and MAT scaled up to 20 percent of opiate-dependent PWID, Pakistan can reduce new infections nationally among PWID by 33 percent compared to a status quo of 2011 levels. This reduction is in the range suggested by previous studies utilizing similar scale-up plans for cities in Pakistan (Strathdee, Hallett et al. 2010). Our scale-up targets are achievable and pragmatic. While Pakistan needs to manage its start-up costs in this vision, it is well within its grasp to achieve high effectiveness for these interventions. As suggested by in-country experts in Pakistan, additional resources and capacities will be required to increase effective coverage, above and beyond current funding and programs via the GFATM and the Government of Pakistan (Pakistan Harm Reduction Technical Advisory Committee 2012).

CHAPTER 5

Thailand Case Study

Overview of the Epidemic

Within Asia, Thailand is one of the only countries with an HIV prevalence close to 1 percent among the adult population (UNAIDS 2010). Much like Thailand's neighbors, however, the Thai HIV epidemic is now concentrated among key populations. In recent reviews of the epidemics among key high-risk groups, the HIV prevalence is estimated to be approximately 23 percent among MSM (Beyrer 2011a) and 11.9 percent among FSW, the latter ranging from 5 percent to 30 percent among direct, in-direct, and street-based sex work (Kerrigan, Wirtz et al. 2012). HIV prevalence is estimated in the range of 30 percent to 40 percent among PWID (UNAIDS 2010). These populations were most affected early in the epidemic, first the MSM and followed by PWID, and peaks in prevalence were observed in the early 1990's. This was followed by a decline, and a resurgence in 1999 (USAID 2010).

Contribution of Injecting Drug Use to the Epidemic

Recent HIV sero-surveillance suggests the national HIV prevalence among PWID remains high and has, in fact, increased from median ranges of 26 percent to 33 percent in 2006–2007 to 48 percent to 52 percent in 2008–2009 (Ministry of Public Health Thailand 2010). Thai estimates of HIV among PWID are variable by geography and sampling method, by which prevalence estimates were reported as 38.6 percent among PWID attending detoxification clinics, while surveillance using respondent-driven sampling in Bangkok and Chiang Mai estimated the HIV prevalence at 23.3 percent and 10.8 percent respectively in 2009 (Ministry of Public Health Thailand 2010).

Figure 5.1   Prevalence Estimates of HIV among Key High-Risk Groups[a]

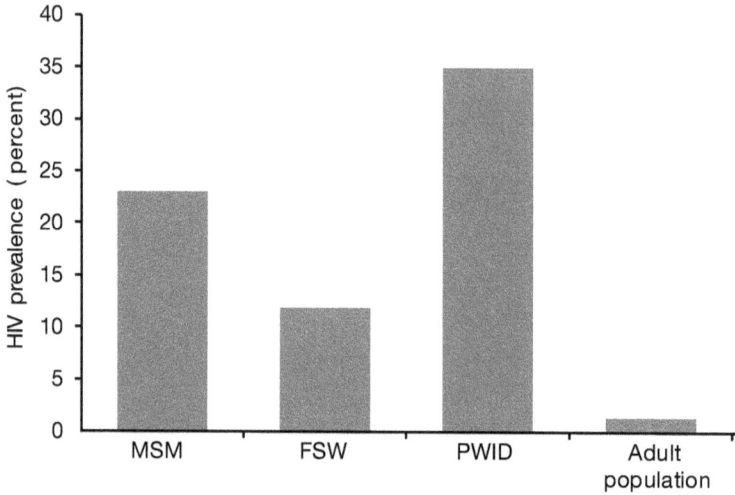

Source: Authors.
Note: FSW = female sex worker; MSM = male sex worker; PWID = people who inject drugs.
a. Estimates of HIV prevalence among FSW are pooled estimates for direct, indirect and
    street-based sex workers.

Modeling estimates from 2009 suggested the incidence was highest among PWID at approximately 2.6 per 100 per year and 0.7 per 100 per year among partners of PWID (Gouws, White et al. 2006b). In 2009, national HIV expenditures estimated that 36 million Thai baht were directed to harm reduction for PWID, representing a total of 4 percent of HIV expenditures despite high incidence and prevalence (Ministry of Public Health Thailand 2010).

Earlier modeling efforts suggested that by 2010, injection drug use would contribute to 9 percent of HIV infections among the adult population in Thailand (The A2 Thailand and the Thai Working Group on HIV/AIDS Projections 2008); given the high prevalence of HIV among the population, it is likely that this is an underestimate of the contribution of injecting drug use to the HIV epidemic. Globally, Thailand is among the ten countries which contribute 70 percent of the global total population of PWID living with HIV (International Harm Reduction Association 2010).

Figure 5.2   HIV Prevalence Estimates among Thai Adult and PWID Populations (1999–2009)

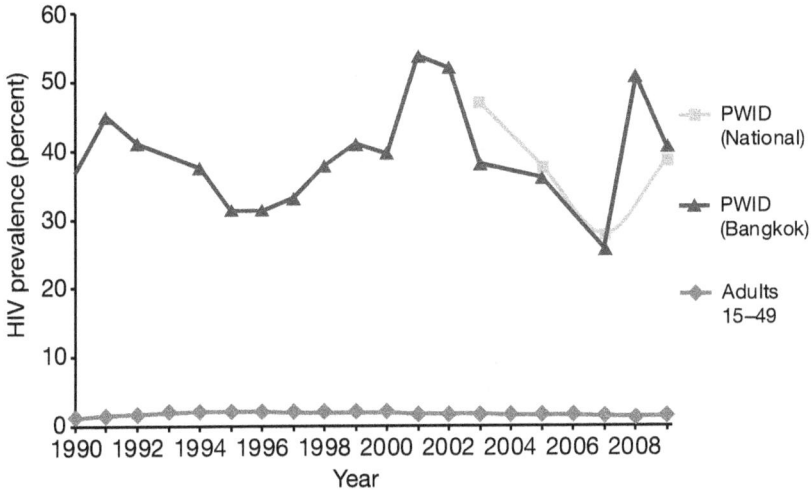

Source: Ministry of Public Health Thailand 2010; UNAIDS 2010.

Heterogeneity of Injecting Drug Use in Thailand

Drug use practices and population characteristics are variable across Thailand. Injecting drug use is commonly associated with, but not limited to, heroin and methamphetamines. Burma remains the world's second largest producer of heroin, and Thailand's principal source for both heroin and methamphetamine. In Bangkok, in addition to heroin (used by approximately 34 percent of PWID), other injected drugs include Midazolam (a benzodiazepine; used by 42 percent of PWID) and yaba (tablet form of methamphetamine; may be a combination of methamphetamine and caffeine) and all of these may also be used in combination and in non-injected forms(Milloy, Fairbairn et al. 2010). Methamphetamines are estimated to be injected by 63 percent of the Bangkok PWID population (Ministry of Public Health Thailand 2010). Methadone (6 percent), dormicum (4 percent), and opium were also injected in Chiang Mai, in addition to heroin (most common: injected by 34 percent) and methamphetamines (32 percent) (Ministry of Public Health Thailand 2010). Drug use begins at a relatively young age (mean 16 yrs.) and BBSS surveys reported that a majority of male and female high school students have used addictive drugs in the past, though predominantly marijuana and methamphetamines. (Ministry of Public Health Thailand 2010)

Increased use of methamphetamines is likely attributable to increased market availability of methamphetamine either in the pill form, yaba, or in crystalline form, in East and Southeast Asia have led to observable increases in use of methamphetamine as well as a 50 percent increase in seizures from 2007 to 2008 and four-fold increase in arrests (Burnett Institute 2010). Much of this increased availability was due to a resurgence of the illicit narcotics economy in neighboring Myanmar, driven by that country's return to ethnic conflict in those years.

The nationwide estimate of needle-sharing is 30 percent; however recent reports findings highlight variations across the country, reporting survey data from Chiang Mai, Songkla, and Samut Prakan that indicate the use of non-sterile equipment by between 26 percent to 64 percent of PWID who were surveyed (Ministry of Public Health Thailand 2010; USAID 2010).

While risk of HIV transmission is often greater within prison settings, risk associated with incarceration in the early part of the decade were particularly great for IDU. An early study from 2001–2002 of 689 male Bangkok prison inmates, demonstrated that 50 percent of the population were PWID and approximately 49 percent of those were actively injecting while in prison. Forty-eight percent of these men reported sharing equipment before and during incarceration, while 21 percent reported initiating sharing during incarceration. HIV incidence among inmates who were actively injecting was estimated to be 11.10 per 100 person years, compared to 4.17 among all inmates. Risks associated with HIV prevalence among all inmates included: history of injection, positive urine opiate test, and history of attendance to drug withdrawal clinics (Thaisri, Lerwitworapong et al. 2003). Similar findings were reported by other studies in northern Thailand (Beyrer, Jittiwutikarn et al. 2003). Most recent estimates from 2009 suggest that 57 percent of incarceration is related to drug-related offences: 18 percent of prisoners were drug users and 82 percent were 'dealers/possessors' of drugs.

While the high-risk injecting practices seem to have declined within the prison system since the early part of the decade, the prevalence of incarcerated people with a history of injecting drug use remains high. Lack of HIV surveillance in the prison system allows for estimation of HIV risk among inmates (Ministry of Public Health Thailand 2010). Other studies report greater risk for overdose associated with incarceration history (Milloy, Fairbairn et al. 2010).

Our case study focuses on HIV outcomes of injecting drug use, however, the prevalence and risk for other infectious disease and health outcomes should not be ignored. PWID in Thailand are great risk for HCV infection (2010 prevalence: 90 percent) and TB (incidence: 142 per 100,000) (International Harm Reduction Association 2010). Overdose as well contributes to a substantial proportion of mortality among PWID. A convenience sample of PWID in Bangkok suggested that almost 30 percent of the population reported a history of non-fatal overdose, predominantly associated with injected heroin, only 30 percent of whom were seen by a healthcare worker. Almost 70 percent reported witnessing an overdose, though only half of participants believed they were capable of preventing or managing an overdose and only 6 percent were knowledgeable of naloxone (Milloy, Fairbairn et al. 2010). Overdose was the leading cause of death of PWID participants in the recent Bangkok Tenofovir Study, with an incidence rate of 0.3 per 100 person-years (95 percent confidence interval 0.2–0.5) (Martin, Vanichseni et al. 2011).

Status of the Four Key Interventions for PWID in Thailand

All key interventions—HCT, NSP, MAT, and ART—exist for PWID in Thailand, though with varying degrees of support and coverage. Historically, there has been limited support for needle and syringe exchange programs and limited substitution therapy for methadone. Currently, NSP does not exist at the national level, thus, in response NGO-run needle exchange programs have developed, approximately 10 sites in 2009 (Burnett Institute 2010) and were accessed by an estimated 413 PWID in a 12-month period (Degenhardt, Mathers et al. 2010). While sterile needles are available for purchase in pharmacies, qualitative research has highlighted the prioritization of PWIDs' personal money towards drug purchases over clean needle purchases (Perngmark, Vanichseni et al. 2008). Despite attempts to increase awareness, needle-sharing practices continue. In response, a coalition of NGOs were successful in seeking non-CCM funding from the Global Fund to provide NSPs, but these programs had difficulty reaching the scale and coverage required to address the needs at national levels in Thailand (Burnett Institute 2010).

MAT sites outnumber NSP, with approximately 134 to 147 sites in operation (Sharma, Oppenheimer et al. 2009; Burnett Institute 2010; Degenhardt, Mathers et al. 2010) and reaching an estimated populations of 4,000 to 5,000 and 150 opioid-dependent people in a 12-month period, via MMT and BMT programs, respectively (Sharma, Oppenheimer et al. 2009; Degenhardt, Mathers et al. 2010). Estimates from 2009 also suggested that approximately 90 compulsory rehabilitation sites and 90 correctional facilities for PWID were operational in Thailand (Degenhardt, Mathers et al. 2010), though such sites are not recommended for HIV prevention or substance use treatment (Jurgens and Csete 2012).

Targeted condom programs and HCT for PWID covered an estimated 15 provinces in 2009, predominantly led by PSI (Burnett Institute 2010). Despite geographic coverage, the range in coverage of PWID who report a history of HIV testing and counseling varies from 36 percent to 71 percent PWID (Kawichai, Celentano et al. 2006; Ministry of Public Health Thailand 2010).

Similarly, the coverage of condom distribution or inclusion within targeted HIV prevention programs for PWID in Thailand is unclear. Condom distribution is important given the risk sexual transmission and low levels of PWID (28.6 percent female and 44.6 percent male) reporting condom use at last sex (UNAIDS 2010).

Modeling Analysis

Model Fitting

The Thailand Goals model was parameterized with data from national sources: HIV incidence until 1990 from UNAIDS AIDSInfo database; PMTCT as well as adult and child ART from the Coverage Survey (2001–2005) and WHO Universal Access Reports (2007– 2010). The HIV prevalence estimates and behavioral data for heterosexual risk groups, MSM, and PWID were inserted into the model and were derived from national estimates presented in UNAIDS and UNGASS reports according to historical trends (Ministry of Public Health Thailand 2010; UNAIDS 2010). Recent reviews for similar reports on MSM and FSW in Thailand also contributed to the historical parameters included in the model (Beyrer 2011a; Kerrigan, Wirtz et al. 2012).

Table 5.1   Model Parameters Related to PWID for the Thailand Case Study

PWID-related parameter	Goals model	Reported estimates	Source
Population size	40,000	40,000 to 178,500	The A2 Thailand and the Thai Working Group on HIV/AIDS Projections 2008; Sharma, Oppenheimer et al. 2009; Mathers, Degenhardt et al. 2010.
Percent using contaminated injecting equipment (all PWID)	43%	26 to 64%	Ministry of Public Health Thailand 2010.
HIV prevalence, male PWID (2009)	38%	38%	UNAIDS 2010.
HIV prevalence, female PWID (2009)	46.2%	46.2%	UNAIDS 2010.
Proportion opiod-dependent	34%	34%[a]	UNAIDS 2010.

Source: Authors; see Source column.
a. Data from Bangkok and Chiang Mai.

Table 5.1 highlights key behavioral and epidemiological inputs for PWID that were used to fit the model. While a recent review of the HIV prevalence among PWID and access to harm reduction by the UN Reference Group suggested the population prevalence of PWID in Thailand is 178,500 (131,500 to 233,000) (Sharma, Oppenheimer et al. 2009; Degenhardt, Mathers et al. 2010), the nationally accepted population size estimate of 40,000 PWID was used for this model (The A2 Thailand and the Thai Working Group on HIV/ AIDS Projections 2008). The model was parameterized with annual epidemiological and behavioral data according to risk group. Table 5.1 presents the most recent reported estimates and sources. As combined, non-gender disaggregated prevalence estimates are often available for the adult population and people who inject drugs, the behavioral and prevalence estimates for the adult population and the PWID populations were applied to male and female PWID when gender-disaggregated data were unavailable.

Adjustments were made to behavioral parameters, when necessary, to achieve a pattern similar to that presented historically. The epidemic curve of the adult population produced by Goals model was checked against national surveillance estimates reported by UNAIDS Country reports (Figure. 5.3), as well as estimated prevalence among PWID (chart not displayed). With the fitted Goals model, a range of coverage levels was applied to these estimates to assess the impact of relevant HIV interventions with varying effectiveness (conservative and optimistic levels of effectiveness as captured in the Goals impact matrix).

Figure 5.3   Comparison of Goals to National Epidemic Curve for HIV in the Adult Population

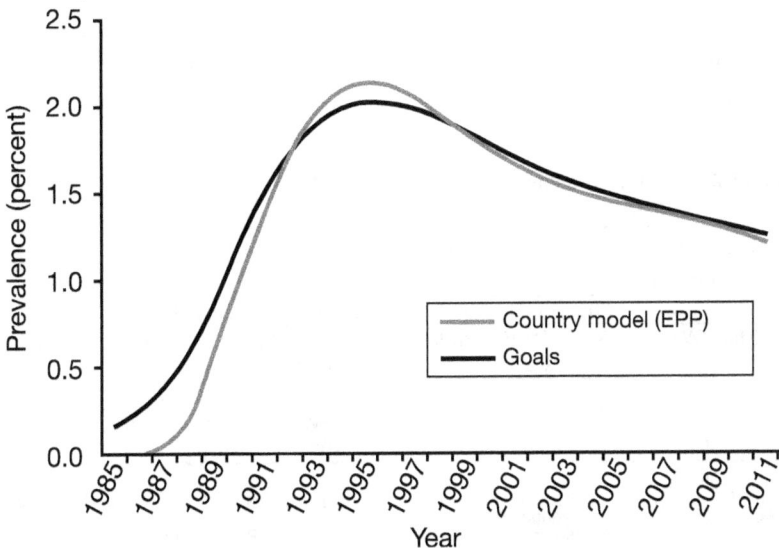

Source: Authors' calculations; UNAIDS.
Note: EPP = estimation and projection package.

Scenarios

Modeling scenarios were described in Chapter 2. We modeled the Status Quo, Baseline, and the two versions of the Expansion scenario. Baseline and the Expansion scenarios were differentiated from each other in terms of the coverage for NSP, MAT, and HCT interventions. Baseline and Expansion scenarios included ART expansion based on Thailand's national estimates of the absolute number of adults in need of ART who receive ART. Unlike behavioral interventions in Goals, ART can be scaled-up only among the overall adult populations, according to CD4 criterion, and cannot be specifically brought to scale among specified risk groups, such as PWID. It is therefore assumed that PWID now achieve a proportionate share in ART coverage, as described in Chapter 2.

The Status Quo was developed to demonstrate the counterfactual scenario for comparison of scaling up interventions for PWID and ART. This scenario projected the number of new infections when all future coverage levels of ART, other adult, other risk population, and PWID interventions were held constant from 2011 levels forward. Baseline (2011) coverage levels of the key prevention interventions were derived from the UN Reference Group reports as well as UNGASS reports and data available on PWID.

Only ART coverage increases in the Baseline scenario. Coverage levels are described in Table 17. In the Baseline scenario, coverage for all key PWID interventions is expected to remain stable over 2011–2015, except for adult ART, to account for national expansion plans.

The epidemic overview presented earlier in this chapter provides a discussion of the history of and current coverage of HIV prevention programs for PWID. Table 5.2 below presents the Status Quo and Baseline coverage estimates.

Table 5.2   Status Quo and Baseline Scenarios for Key Interventions among PWID in Thailand

Intervention	2011	2012	2013	2014	2015
ART: status quo	205,415				
ART: baseline	205,415	209,504	216,612	221,448	224,388
HCT for PWID[c]	39% of PWID (Kawichai, Celentano et al. 2006; Ministry of Health Ukraine 2010; Ministry of Public Health Thailand 2010)				
NSP[c]	1% of all PWID[a] (Degenhardt, Mathers et al. 2010)				
MAT[c]	32%[b] of all opioid-dependent PWID (Degenhardt, Mathers et al. 2010)				

Source: Authors.
Note: ART = antiretroviral therapy; HCT = HIV counseling and testing; MAT = medically assisted therapy; NSP = needle and syringe program.
a. Authors' calculations based on number PWID accessing NSP/ PWID population of 40,000
b. Authors' calculations based on number PWID accessing MAT/ opioid dependent population
c. Coverage level held constant across years for status quo and baseline scenarios

In the Baseline scenario, coverage levels for HCT, NSP, and MAT are maintained over 2012–2015 as in the table above. The Goals model was run for the Status Quo and Baseline scenarios and uncertainty analysis was conducted.

Table 2.1 in Chapter 2 described the scale-up ranges proposed in the WHO/UNODC/UNAIDS Technical Guide. According to this guidance, we established an expansion path from 2012–2015 for Thailand for the four key interventions. The choice of the final endpoint in 2015 for coverage was based on an estimate of what was the appropriate target given current coverage, and what was needed. Based on 2011 coverage levels, we thus aimed to increase coverage of NSP from "Low" to "Medium" and increase coverage of MAT and HCT from "Medium" to "High" targeted coverage.

For NSP, we set the target as 40 percent coverage of all PWID, which is in the "Medium" range from the guide. We assumed a linear expansion path from current 2011 coverage to this value over the four years 2012–2015. For MAT, we set a scale-up target of 60 percent of opioid-dependent people by 2015, drawing from the "High" range of the technical guide. Because there is no separate entry for opioid-dependent PWID in the Goals model, the scale-up of MAT was reflected within Goals by a scale-up from 0.11 to 0.2 percent of the total population of PWID. For HCT, we set a target of 75 percent of PWID from the "High" range. The results are listed in Table 5.3 for the Expansion scenarios.

Table 5.3   Expansion Scenario Coverage for the Four Key Interventions among PWID in Thailand

Intervention	2011	2012	2013	2014	2015
ART	205,415	209,504	216,612	221,448	224,388
HCT for PWID	39%	48%	57%	66%	75%
NSP	1%	11%	21%	30%	40%
MAT	32%	43%	54%	64%	75%

Source: Authors.
Note: ART = antiretroviral therapy; HCT = HIV counseling and testing; MAT = medically assisted therapy; NSP = needle and syringe program.

Results

Figure 5.4 projects the epidemic curve of new HIV infections among PWID in Thailand from 2011 through 2015. In the absence of any HIV intervention expansion, including ART, an increasing number of new infections among PWID is observed (depicted by Status Quo). Allowing the estimated expansion of ART to occur among the adult population and, thus, among PWID, substantially changes the epidemic trajectory among PWID (Baseline). The additional expansion of the key interventions, as depicted by both Expansion scenarios, elicits further reductions in new infections among PWID, with greatest improvements observed with the optimistic effectiveness in expansion (Expansion Optimistic).

Figure 5.4   New HIV Infections among PWID in Thailand Compared across Modeled Scenarios

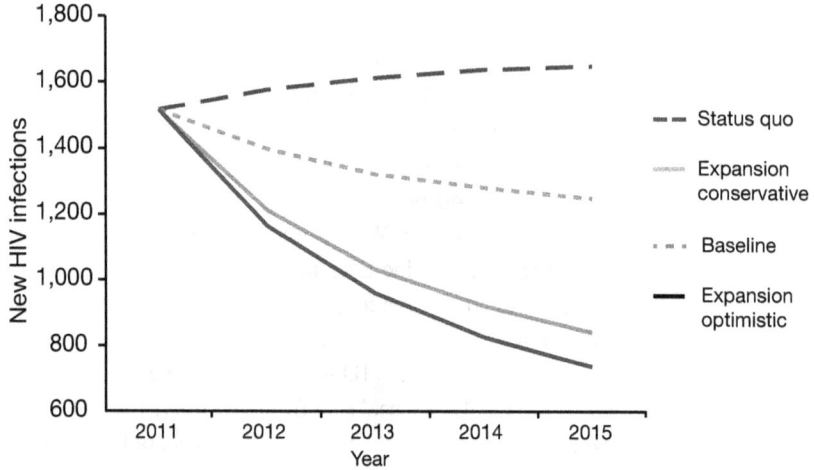

Source: Authors' calculations.

HIV transmission among the overall adult population is affected by scale-up of these interventions as well. Table 5.4 present a comparison of the number of infections averted among the adult population with these expansion scenarios.

Table 5.4   Averted HIV Infections among Adults 15–49 Years Old in Thailand, by Modeled Scenario

Year	Compared to status quo		Compared to baseline	
	Baseline	Expansion optimistic	Expansion conservative	Expansion optimistic
2012	2,908	3,139	184	231
2013	4,671	5,036	290	365
2014	5,451	5,905	360	454
2015	5,822	6,340	411	518
Overall	18,852	20,420	1,245	1,568

Source: Authors.

Comparing the Baseline and Expansion Optimistic interventions to Status Quo, we can demonstrate the benefits observed with the proportionate availability of ART to PWID in treatment expansion (Baseline) and then the addition of expanded and highly effective coverage of the three other key PWID interventions (Expansion Optimistic). From 2012 to 2015 almost 18,900 infections among adults are averted with proportionate access in ART expansion. If the expansion of key PWID HIV interventions is added with ART expansion it provides additional benefits compared to Status Quo, resulting in a cumulative 20,400 infections averted.

Comparing the Expansion scenarios to Baseline can address questions similar to those raised in previous case studies for Ukraine and Pakistan. Is it worthwhile to add scale-up in terms of a combination prevention package? In this case, almost 1,250 infections may be averted among adults with additional expansion of NSP, MAT, and HCT over and above ART; and 1,570 infections may be averted if these interventions are highly effective.

Table 5.5   Incremental Cost-Effectiveness Ratios, US$ per Averted Adult Infection, Thailand

Year	Compared to status quo		Compared to baseline	
	Baseline	Expansion optimistic	Expansion conservative	Expansion optimistic
2012	$291	$557	$4,900	$3,903
2013	$306	$630	$6,016	$4,774
2014	$447	$842	$7,063	$5,588
2015	$499	$977	$8,031	$6,352
Overall	$404	$788	$6,819	$5,403

Source: Authors.

Inspection of total costs associated with ART expansion alone, suggests an additional US$7.6 million will be spent during this time period (comparing Baseline costs to Status Quo). Compared to the Baseline, expansion of key interventions among PWID will cost an additional US$8.5 million. Using total costs associated with the scale-up of these interventions, the ICER are presented in Table 5.5.

Uncertainty Analysis

Concluding the analysis, we ran 500 iterations for each scenario, varying the impact matrix parameters and unit costs, resulting in distributions for various model outputs. We recorded the medians and the 95 percent confidence intervals for new HIV infections and total costs for each scenario. Comparing scenarios, Figure 5.5 displays the possible range in ICER based on infections averted. The uncertainty analysis suggests that depending on the parameters chosen, Thailand may see expansion of NSP, MAT, and HCT for PWID over and above expanding ART as being very cost-effective to just cost-effective, given a scenario lower impact of the interventions (i.e., conservative impact matrix). Other conclusions from above are unchanged, especially when interventions are highly impactful.

Figure 5.5   Overall ICER for Thailand Scenarios 2012–15: Median, 95 Percent CI

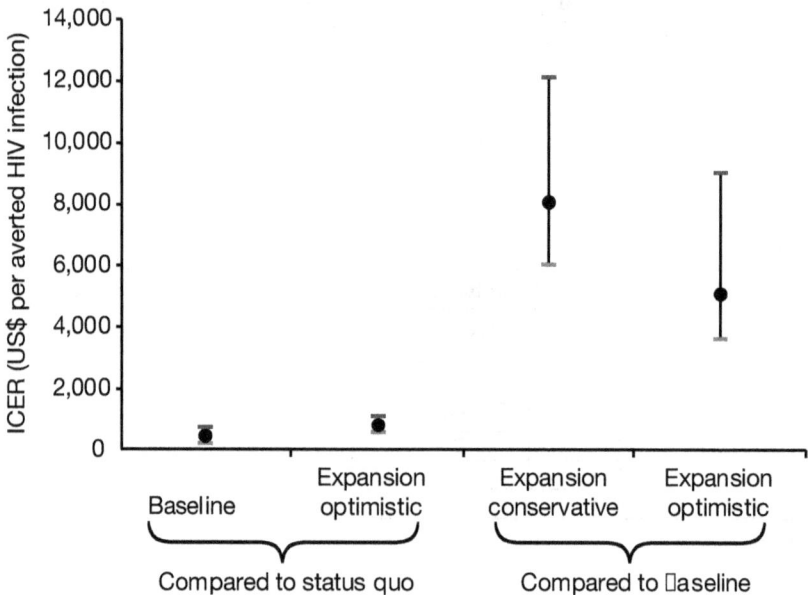

Source: Authors.
Note: ICER = incremental cost-effectiveness ratio

Discussion

Well into the HIV epidemic and despite knowledge of the high HIV prevalence among PWID in Thailand, HIV prevention programs for PWID remain low, particularly for NSP. These historical trends affect programming for PWID and likely play a critical role in the overall epidemic among PWID and general population and late changes to health policy may suggest the possibility of a changed epidemic trajectory.

In 2003 the "War on Drugs" policy of the Thai government was instituted and, though no longer continued, it has left a lasting effect on HIV prevention for PWID. Residual stigma, discrimination and violence toward PWID, as well as fear on the part of PWID, continue to act as barriers in efforts of NGOs to provide services and PWID to access services. As of 2010, only 10 NSP sites were operational and were reportedly run by NGOs who continued to face operational and political challenges and risk police crackdowns (International Harm Reduction Association 2010).

The National AIDS Plan for 2007–2011 aimed to reduce HIV incidence among PWID by half during this period; this plan generally included stigma/ discrimination reduction, surveillance and research, and outreach to PWID in the community and detention centers (Ministry of Public Health Thailand 2010). Harm reduction has been made explicit in national policy documents and needle exchange programs and opioid substitution programs are operational, although, NSPs are not supported by the government (Burnett Institute 2010; International Harm Reduction Association 2010). Methadone programs have been included in the National Healthcare Scheme as of 2008 (Ministry of Public Health Thailand 2010) with further expansion of these services supported by Round 8 of the Global Fund (AHRN 2009).

This study demonstrates the impact on HIV incidence among the PWID and overall adult populations in Thailand from the scale-up of four key harm reduction interventions. We observed significant declines in new infections when ART expands among the adult population and proportionate access to ART is allowed for PWID. Among PWID, these interventions result in a cumulative 35 percent reduction in new infections. These benefits in averting new infections are enhanced with the addition of key interventions for PWID. The benefits to the adult population can also not be ignored, among whom 5,000 to 6,000 new infections were averted over the four-year period. One cannot assume that ART expansion will mean access for PWID. There is limited knowledge of the coverage of ART among PWID in Thailand, while some studies suggest access to ART for PWID living with HIV/AIDS is minimal at best.

As findings emerge presenting the benefits of ART as prevention, and the cost of ART drugs declines, scale-up of ART for PWID will be both equitable and feasible. Currently, the Bangkok Tenofovir Study, a double-blind placebo controlled trial among HIV negative PWID (N = 2413) is underway to assess the use of oral tenofovir for the prevention of HIV transmission and may demonstrate further use of ART drugs for prevention of transmission among PWID (Martin, Vanichseni et al. 2011).

Several limitations should be taken into consideration when interpreting the results we have presented. First, we used a national population size estimate of 40,000 PWID for Thailand. However, there is a broad range of estimates reported for PWID, spanning from 40,000 to 178,500. If the population size is closer to the high end of the range, the incidence, coverage achieved, and cost-effectiveness results may be biased. Second, in relying on surveillance and published data, this modeling effort may be limited by reporting biases. Changes in the number of MAT or NSP sites may not yet be captured and behavioral data, predominantly captured in urban settings may not be generalizable to other areas of Thailand. Finally, while condom provision is considered with our modeling exercise, the relationship of sexual transmission among PWID and non-PWID is limited within Goals.

The four key harm reduction interventions not only have a place in the general Thai society but can serve an important role to address risks in the incarcerated setting as well. Earlier we highlighted the transmission risks within the prison and detention facilities are a significant source of drug rehabilitation and treatment as well as HIV prevention, if implemented properly and without coercions. Though not included in this model, these environments should not be overlooked in their potential impact on the HIV epidemic, social contexts, and lives of Thai PWID. However, focus first should be placed on creating alternatives to incarceration for PWID. Recent legislation suggests Thailand may be moving in this direction, with voluntary rehabilitation of PWID, treating them as patients as opposed to criminals and moving 20 percent of drug-related offenders from prison each year (Rouanvong 2007).

Finally, other interventions to reduce harm to PWID may be considered. First, though predominantly underground, naloxone programs have been initiated in response to the drug overdose death rate of 8.97 per 1,000 person years among HIV-negative PWID in Thailand (Quan, Vongchak et al. 2007; International Harm Reduction Association 2010; Milloy, Fairbairn et al. 2010). Given the high prevalence of HBV, HCV, and TB, a comprehensive approach will involve additional measures to prevent and treat such co-infections among PWID living with HIV.

Full access to and utilization of services cannot be achieved without realization of rights for people who inject drugs. Thailand's historical War on Drugs, current criminal sanctions, and resulting harassment and arrest by law enforcement perpetuate the underground nature of drug use. While Thailand appears to be changing the attitude towards PWID for the better, for example by the 2002 Narcotics Rehabilitation Act recognizes PWID as patients rather than criminals, true uptake and implementation has been questionable. These issues impede the provision of harm reduction services offered by NGOs, the access to these services by PWID, and proper surveillance and evaluations of existing service. Thus, vulnerability and low coverage levels of services for PWID may be perpetuated in Thailand (Burnett Institute 2010).

CHAPTER 6

Kenya Case Study

Overview of the Epidemic

Kenya has a population of 39 million people and remains the largest economy in East Africa with a GDP of nearly US$30 billion as compared to approximately US$21 billion in Tanzania and US$16 billion in Uganda. The first case of HIV was estimated to have occurred in 1978 with the first AIDS case officially reported in 1984 (Kawewa 2005). The first and most clearly identified risk factor related to HIV infection at that time was sex work (Kawewa 2005). By 1986, 286 cases had been observed with 38 AIDS-related deaths. The epidemic became generalized in the coming years and sentinel surveillance systems demonstrated prevalence of 5.1 percent by 1990, peaking at 13.4 percent in 2000 (Kimani, Kaul et al. 2008). As of 2009, Kenya had approximately 1.5 million people (range 1.3–1.6 million) living with HIV, of which 1.3 million (1.2–1.4 million) are reproductive age adults between 15–49 years. Today the generalized epidemic has stabilized, and new surveillance findings suggest Kenya has a mixed epidemic (NACC and NASCOP 2011).

Since 2000, there has been a decline in estimated HIV prevalence in the general population with current prevalence estimated at approximately 6.3 percent among adults which is slightly lower than the 7 percent which was observed in the Kenyan AIDS Indicator Survey in 2003 and 8.4 percent reported in 2001 (Cheluget, Baltazar et al. 2006). These declines are especially apparent in urban sites and have corresponded with reductions in higher-risk sexual practices in the general population, the scale-up of ART, and better data through improved HIV surveillance (UNAIDS 2005; UNAIDS 2008). About 760,000 women 15 years and older are estimated to be living with HIV as of 2009 representing about 58 percent of all infections among adults (UNAIDS 2010). HIV prevalence was observed to be almost twice as high among females as among males, with an estimated 8 percent of reproductive age women living with HIV as compared to 4 percent among men. The disproportionate burden of HIV among women in Kenya has remained consistent throughout the history of the epidemic.

There is considerable geographic heterogeneity within the HIV epidemic in Kenya. Nyanza province has the highest prevalence at 13.9 percent which is approximately twice the prevalence of the next highest (7 percent in Nairobi and Western provinces). In comparison, less than one percent of adults are living with HIV in Northeastern province.

Understanding the Mixed Epidemic in Kenya

The 2011 UNGASS report for Kenya highlighted the heighted risk and prevalence among Kenya's key high-risk populations, particularly FSW and FSW clients, MSM, PWID and prisoners. This same report suggested that inadequate surveillance methods allow for insufficient understanding of HIV prevalence among key populations (NACC and NASCOP 2011).

Figure 6.1   Prevalence Estimates of HIV among Key High-Risk Groups

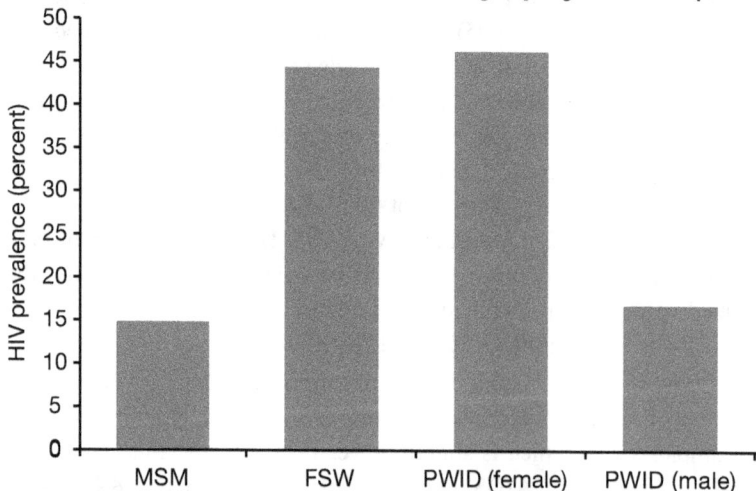

Source: Beyrer 2011b; Kerrigan, Wirtz et al. 2012; UNODC 2012.
Note: FSW = female sex worker; MSM = male sex worker; PWID = people who inject drugs.

A Modes of Transmission analysis was completed in 2008 which estimated sources of new infections (NACC and World Bank 2009). The largest source of new infections was estimated to be heterosexual sex within union or with regular partners, contributing 44 percent of new infections, followed by heterosexual sex with casual partners, or multiple partnerships. Men who have sex with men and prisoners were estimated to contribute 15 percent of new infections, and sex work contributed 14 percent. Injecting drug use was estimated to contribute 3.8 to 4.8 percent of new infections (Beaveau 2006).

Previous reviews commissioned by the World Bank have thus investigated the prevalence in key high-risk populations, demonstrating that although HIV has declined among the general population, infection remains high among MSM and FSW (Beyrer 2011b; Kerrigan, Wirtz et al. 2012). Figure 6.1 provides a comparison of levels.

Injecting Drug Use in Kenya

People who use drugs including PWID are increasingly recognized as an at-risk population in Kenya (Ndetei 2004; Gouws, White et al. 2006a; Singh, Brodish et al. 2011). A recent rapid situational analysis (RSA) of PWID in Nairobi and Coast provinces highlights the high HIV prevalence among PWID (Figure 6.1), ranging from 17 percent to 47 percent among male and female PWID, respectively (UNODC 2012).

The use of several drugs has been reported including injected cocaine (UNODC 2012), *bhangi, khat, benzodiazepines*, glue, and alcohol (Strathdee, Hallett et al. 2010; Geibel et al. 2011). Studies in Nairobi and Coast Province suggest that almost 98 percent of the PWID population inject heroin (Tun, Okal et al. 2011; UNODC 2012). While white and brown heroin are used, white heroin has been the most common initiator drug of choice (Geibel et al. 2011).

A UNODC study in 2004 found that 80 percent of injectors in three urban centers reported sharing injection devices, with 50 percent being HIV positive in the coastal city of Mombasa. In a WHO study in Nairobi, HIV prevalence was 53 percent among PWID, two-thirds of whom also reported sexual risks (Odek-Ogunde 2004). Access to harm reduction services is limited as public clinics do not provide medically-assisted therapy (Mathers, Degenhardt et al. 2010; Strathdee, Hallett et al. 2010).

The recent RSA study provides substantial information on the high risk practices among PWID. The study included a sample of 540 PWID in Nairobi and the Coast Province, 91 percent of whom were male and mostly between the ages of 15 to 34 years (UNODC 2012). High-risk injecting practices were common with nearly 40 percent sharing needles/syringes; less than 20 percent had accessed drug dependence treatment (UNODC 2012).

Other studies have reported similar findings, and elaborated the high risk practices among Nairobi PWID. Among HIV positive PWID, 61 percent reported lending a used needle, 66 percent reported using front or back-loaded syringes, and 60 percent reported drawing drugs from a common container within the last month (Tun, Okal et al. 2011). Injecting frequency was daily for approximately 80 percent of the PWID population, 75 percent reporting at least two injections per day (Geibel et al. 2011), and needles were reused approximately five times prior to disposal (Tun, Okal et al. 2011). HIV prevalence was 19.6 percent (adjusted) though there was great geographic variability with 27.7 percent HIV prevalence in Nairobi and 3.3 percent in coastal Kilifi, and there was marked gender variation (UNODC 2012).

Risky sexual behavior related to PWID in Kenya cannot be overlooked. Forty percent of the PWID population surveyed in Nairobi was sexually active in the month prior to survey, with 30 percent reporting unprotected sex acts. Approximately 30 percent of PWID reported more than one sexual partner in the last year (Geibel et al. 2011). High-risk sexual practices were common with 20 percent reporting transactional sex, and only 40 percent reporting condom use during sex (UNODC 2012). Violence was also prevalent: 20 percent of those interviewed in Nairobi reported physical violence in the last year and 1 percent reported sexual violence in the last year (Geibel et al. 2011).

Drug overdose was also common among Nairobi and Coastal PWID: 86 percent of PWID reported witnessing an overdose, 58 percent knew someone who had died of an overdose; and 37 percent of PWID had personally experienced a non-fatal overdose at least once, yet understanding of management and response to overdose was not common among PWID (UNODC 2012). Finally, 81 percent of this population reported a history of incarceration and seven percent reported injecting drugs while in prison with concurrent needle-sharing practices (UNODC 2012). Given overcrowding, violence, high prevalence of HIV-related risk behaviors, and lack of HIV prevention programs for prisoners, such risk for the PWID population is important to address (UNODC 2007).

Status of HIV Prevention Among PWID in Kenya

The national response to the HIV epidemic has mainly focused on heterosexual partnerships and vertical transmission from mother to child although there has recently been increased attention to key populations (NASCOP 2009). In 2009, the Kenyan National AIDS Council launched the third Kenya National AIDS Strategic Plan (KNASP-III) (NASCOP 2009). The KNASP-III includes a significant component of prevention focused on key high-risk populations, reflecting the increased understanding of a burden of HIV among these populations.

As part of its response, Kenya has adopted the third edition of the antiretroviral drug therapy treatment program that includes free treatment. As of November 2011, 535,121 people living with HIV were on treatment (91 percent were adults or 486,960). While the most recent publicly available guidelines suggest a CD4 threshold of 200 cells per mm^3, new guidelines defining a threshold of 350 cells per mm3 are being adopted and operationalized. There is no evidence that a significant number of PWID received ART as of 2011—the number is expected to be below 200 (Kenya IDU TWG 2011).

Injecting drug use is illegal in Kenya and the lack of legal framework to support the provision of services for the users combined with criminalization and policies which have marginalized the PWID population, access to prevention and treatment services has been greatly inhibited (NACC and NASCOP 2011). Partners in Kenya are engaged in advocacy and sensitization with the legal establishment to address this. Historically, none of the key interventions for PWID except ART, such as NSP and MAT, were officially allowed. Despite this some services were provided by NGO over the last five years, but on a small scale and without legal protection. The NGO include the following from Coast Province with differing areas of operation. Based on data provided at a recent meeting in Nairobi (Kenya IDU TWG 2011), the Omari Project served 2,063 PWID and the Reachout Centre Trust served 5,005 PWID over 2008–11. In Nairobi province, the Nairobi Outreach Services Trust or NOSET provided services to 6,721 PWID over 2005–2010. None of these services included MAT, and reach of NSP was marginal at best. The NGO mainly concentrated on rehabilitation, abscess and overdose treatment, detoxification, and counseling.

Despite these activities, the recent Nairobi respondent-driven sampling study suggested limited exposure of PWID to these locations and services. Less than one-third had received any services in the last year; and when received, the majority utilized abscess treatment and outpatient counseling, which would not prevent HIV transmission. Changes are on the horizon as GFATM Round 10 funding support will help to provide harm reduction activities at a few sites utilizing the NGO.

Modeling Analysis

Model Fitting

Kenya's projection was calibrated with data from the RSA study in PWID in Nairobi and Coast provinces, baseline assessment and size estimation of key high-risk groups in Nairobi, and from the National AIDS and STI Control Program (NASCOP) estimates. Many of these sources were described above in the Overview of the Epidemic. As mentioned above, the estimates of HIV prevalence among PWID in the 2002–2009 timeframe range from around 30 percent to 50 percent.

Figure 6.2   Comparison of Goals to National Epidemic Curve for HIV in the Adult Population

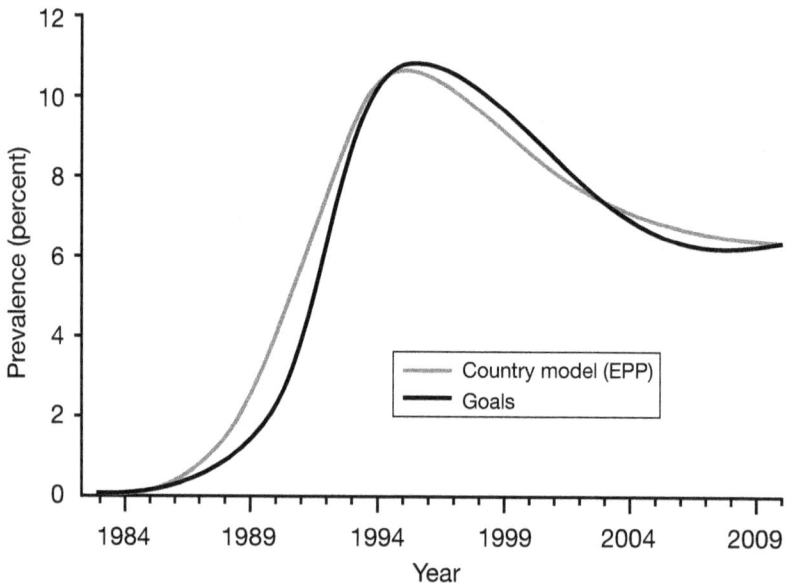

Source: Authors.
Note: EPP = estimation and projection package.

As discussed in Chapter 2, size estimation as a percentage of the adult 15–49 years old population is required for each risk group modeled in Goals. A key focus for this discussion is the size of the PWID population nationally. Studies suggest that there are more PWID in Coast (19,720) than the Nairobi province (11,700). The approximate total may be 31,420 in these two regions

(UNODC 2012). Other studies suggest the proportion of PWID in Kenya from 0.1 percent to 1 percent of the adult population, with 10 percent of injectors estimated to be women (Geibel 2011). Those estimates would lead to much higher figures. We used a population estimated of 35,000 PWID in Kenya, slightly higher than the UNODC estimate across the two key provinces, to account for other PWID who may reside outside Nairobi or Coast provinces. It is important to note that little is known of such PWID.

Scenarios

The Status Quo scenario assumes prevention programs are not scaled up. Baseline scenario allows for increasing coverage of ART among the adult population, as per the national strategy and it assumes that PWID in need of ART have equi-proportionate access to ART. The other key interventions (NSP, MAT, and HCT for PWID) remain at their current levels, per program documentation. Table 6.1 presents the coverage for the Status Quo and Baseline scenarios.

Table 6.1   Status Quo and Baseline Scenarios for Key Interventions among PWID in Kenya

Intervention	2011	2012	2013	2014	2015
ART: status quo[a]			460,867		
ART: baseline	460,867	572,929	669,999	732,558	766,020
HCT for PWID			10% of PWID		
NSP			1% of PWID		
MAT[b]			1% of opioid-dependent PWID		

Source: Authors.
Note: ART = antiretroviral therapy; HCT = HIV counseling and testing; MAT = medically assisted therapy; NSP = needle and syringe program.
a. Mid-year estimate based on percent of HIV-positive adults on ART given current eligibility thresholds.
b. 98 percent of the PWID population is estimated to be opioid-dependent.

The Expansion scenarios represent a case in which programs are extended from their current levels to reach 20 percent of PWID with NSP, MAT, and HCT among PWID. Given that programs are just beginning in Kenya, we chose targets from the "Low" range of the technical guide—see Table 6.1. The scale-up of MAT was assumed to increase from 1 percent to 20 percent of the total population of opioid-dependent PWID. Table 6.2 below displays the estimated increase in coverage levels.

Table 6.2   Expansion Scenario Coverage for the Four Key Interventions among PWID in Kenya

Intervention	2011	2012	2013	2014	2015
ART	460,867	572,929	669,999	732,558	766,020
HCT for PWID	10%	12.5%	15%	17.5%	20%
NSP	10%	12.5%	15%	17.5%	20%
MAT	1%	5.8%	10.5%	15.3%	20%

Source: Authors.
Note: ART = antiretroviral therapy; HCT = HIV counseling and testing; MAT = medically assisted therapy; NSP = needle and syringe program.

Results

With no increase in the services being offered to PWID, we would expect to continue to see an increase in new infections during this time period (i.e., the Status Quo). Offering equi-proportionate access to ART as that intervention is expanded among adults should change the trajectory of the epidemic among PWID (Baseline). This is what we observe; the comparison of Status Quo to Baseline reveals that proportionate access helps to avert approximately 900 new HIV infections in Kenyan PWID between 2012 and 2015.

Figure 6.3   New HIV Infections among PWID in Kenya by Year and Scenario

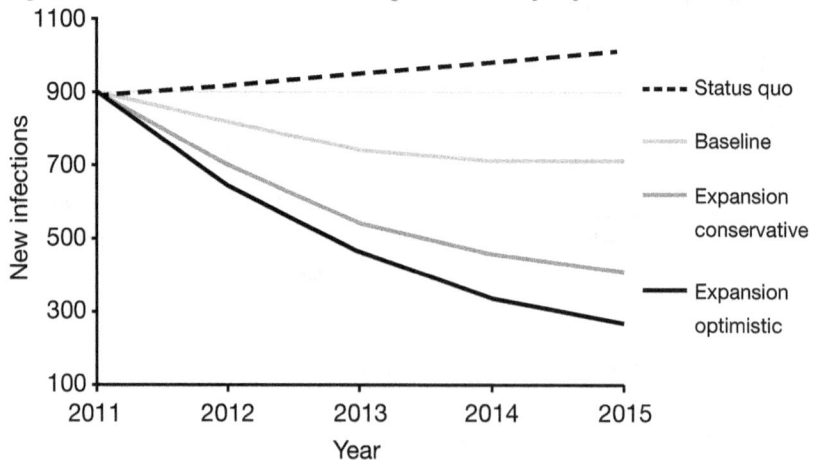

Source: Authors.

As Figure 6.3 demonstrates, the additional expansion of expansion of PWID interventions (Expansion scenarios) adds to the benefits observed with increased ART, as new HIV infections are further reduced in this population, particularly with the expansion of highly effective NSP, MAT, and HCT for PWID (Expansion Optimistic). Compared to Status Quo, this maximally effective package for PWID would avert almost 2,180 new infections among PWID in Kenya over 2012–2015.

Due to mixing of sexual and injecting networks, HIV transmission among the overall adult population should also be affected by scale-up of PWID-specific interventions, and the scale-up of ART has its independent effect. This is described in Table 6.3.

Table 6.3   Averted HIV Infections Among Adults 15–49 Years Old in Kenya, by Modeled Scenario

Year	Compared to status quo		Compared to baseline	
	Baseline	Expansion optimistic	Expansion conservative	Expansion optimistic
2012	10,943	11,120	121	177
2013	24,164	24,448	193	284
2014	32,902	33,271	250	369
2015	36,769	37,224	308	455
Overall	104,778	106,063	872	1,285

Source: Authors.

Comparing the Baseline and Expansion Optimistic interventions to Status Quo we can demonstrate the benefits observed with the introduction of proportionate access to ART expansion (Baseline) and then the addition of a combination prevention package of effective PWID interventions (Expansion Optimistic). From 2012 to 2015 almost 104,778 HIV infections among adults are averted with scaling up ART alone and providing equitable access, compared to flat-lining interventions. Including the expansion of key PWID HIV interventions with ART scale-up provides a moderate increase, resulting in a cumulative 106,063 infections averted.

Specifically, what incremental benefit does the additional scale-up of NSP, MAT, and HCT really provide? Note that ART scales up in both worlds, and the only difference is the scale-up of the other three interventions. Comparing the two Expansion scenarios to Baseline we find that in this case, approximately 870 HIV infections may be averted among adults with further expansion of t hree PWID interventions and approximately 1,300 may be averted if these are highly effective. As Kenya is a mixed epidemic, this may not seem to be a significant large proportion of new infections; however, if we were to carry this analysis over further years, the impact could be greater.

Policy and programming decisions in a resource-limited mixed epidemic rely on selecting interventions that may reduce HIV transmission while being cost-effective. Additional costs related to expansion of ART as suggested in Table 6.2, compared to Status Quo will reach US$153 million. The addition of highly effective PWID interventions alongside ART expansion would cost an additional US$170 million over Status Quo. With inspection we can see that the difference is the additional cost of expansion of NSP, MAT, and HCT for PWID, which is approximately US$17 million, the same as the difference in costs between Baseline and Expansion scenarios.

Conducting an incremental cost-effectiveness analysis, we assessed the cost-effectiveness of these expanded PWID interventions. The ICER for this are presented in Table 6.4.

Table 6.4   Incremental Cost-Effectiveness Ratios, US$ per Averted Adult Infection, Kenya

Year	Compared to status quo		Compared to baseline	
	Baseline	Expansion optimistic	Expansion conservative	Expansion optimistic
2012	$1,920	$2,049	$14,674	$10,031
2013	$1,511	$1,636	$18,018	$12,243
2014	$1,386	$1,524	$20,368	$13,793
2015	$1,351	$1,512	$21,371	$14,453
Overall	$1,459	$1,600	$19,412	$13,166

Source: Authors.

Compared to flat-lining interventions, the scale-up of proportionate ART among adults (Baseline), as well as the combined scale-up of ART and PWID intervention (Expansion Optimistic) have ICER of about US$1,500 to $1,600 based on infections averted. Kenya's 2011 GNI per capita at purchasing power parity was US$1,680 (World Bank 2010). If WHO-CHOICE criteria are applied to the situation–given caveats expressed in Chapter 2—Kenyan policymakers may find this affordable.

Focusing on comparing the two Expansion scenarios to Baseline, the overall ICER across the period ranged from $13,160 to $19,400. Applying previous criteria, it appears that scaling up NSP, MAT, and HCT for PWID over and above equi-proportionate access to scaled-up ART is not cost-effective in Kenya. These three interventions are averting only a moderate number of infections in addition (Table 6.3), while additional costs are US$17 million. As programs scale-up for harm reduction, unit costs will decline with greater economies of scale. The Kenyan combination harm reduction strategy is in its infancy and there are significant start-up and capacity building costs. It is also possible that greater reduction in adult infections may be seen from these interventions if the sexual mixing between PWID and other risk groups is modeled more extensively, though this is uncertain. If this channel has a significant effect, then we may find that expanding PWID-specific interventions is cost-effective.

What is critical to observe from these results is that compared to the current situation of low to absent coverage, a combination package of harm reduction interventions implemented at high effectiveness is very cost-effective (ICER of US$1,600). This is the real consideration for Kenya at this point when it attempts to address the complex needs among PWID, including non-HIV health risks such as overdose and psychosocial conditions.

Uncertainty Analysis

Concluding the analysis, we ran 500 iterations for each scenario, varying the impact matrix parameters and unit costs, resulting in distributions for various model outputs. We recorded the medians and the 95 percent plausibility intervals for new HIV infections and total costs for each scenario.

Figure 6.4 Overall ICER for Kenya Scenarios 2012–15: Median, 95 Percent Confidence Intervals

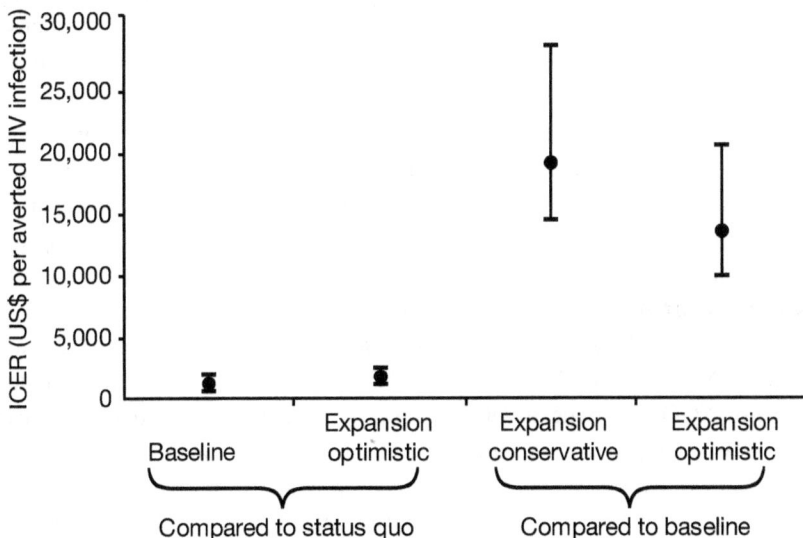

Comparing scenarios, Figure 6.4 displays the possible range in ICER based on infections averted. The results corroborate our findings above, and add strength to our finding that a combination package of harm reduction interventions combining NSP, MAT, HCT, and ART for PWID can be very cost-effective compared to the current low coverage status quo. This is not affected by variability in impact and unit cost parameters.

Discussion

Emerging data suggest a mixed epidemic in Kenya: while HIV prevalence has stabilized among approximately 6 percent among the adult population, it is even greater among key populations at higher risk. The HIV prevalence among PWID has been reported in ranges of 20 percent to 50 percent, driven by high levels of risky injection practices and other risk, and low coverage of harm reduction aimed at HIV prevention.

We have presented a model-based analysis of the scale-up of PWID key interventions, increasing these from a current low or absence of coverage situation. Modeling the impact of key interventions for PWID, including HCT, NSP, and MAT, alongside expansion of ART among the adult population in need of ART, we observe impacts among both the PWID population and the adult population. Equi-proportionate access to ART alone demonstrates that approximately 900 infections may be averted. Expanding highly effective PWID services in combination with ART could avert over 2,000 new infections among PWID between 2012 and 2015, a 56 percent reduction compared to a Status Quo scenario.

There are strong indications that the status quo will not persevere. The GFATM Round 10 grant, which has two Principal Recipients in the Kenya Red Cross and NASCOP, plans to reach a number of PWID through harm reduction interventions over the next few years. Interventions include drop-in NSP centers that will be progressively rolled-out with training of site-level workers. Current plans call for reaching 3,125 PWID in Coast and Nairobi provinces, as well as in Nakuru district (Rift Valley Province) and Kisumu district (Nyanza Province) (Kenya IDU TWG 2011). Sub-recipients include some of NGO experienced with providing outreach and outpatient services to PWID, and hence it is expected that this program can rapidly become successful. This is a welcome development in East Africa, and it follows the experience of scaling up harm reduction in neighboring Tanzania. However, structural changes are also required in the region.

Several limitations should be considered when interpreting these results. First, this model relied on reported data of the PWID population in Kenya.

Recent research has led to increased knowledge of the PWID population, yet most studies are conducted in Nairobi or the Coast and capture predominantly male populations. As a result, several questions remain:

1. What is the true population size of PWID in Kenya?

2. Are the risks observed via surveillance generalizable to the entire PWID population?

3. How do the key interventions affect overdose-related mortality which is considered to be important?

4. How much do risk groups overlap and can targeted prevention programs be synergized for maximum efficiency and increased cost-effectiveness?

As surveillance and research continue, we expect that further analyses of this population may emerge and inform the development of related HIV- and overdose-prevention programs.

Recognizing the high prevalence of HIV infection among PWID and their sexual overlap with other risk groups, experts would suggest that acting to halt the transmission while it is concentrated within this population is urgent to prevent further increases in the HIV epidemic. Programs such as HCT, NSP, and condom distribution for PWID could be coupled with existing outreach programs, and may be overlapped with outreach programs which target FSW, given the level of drug use among this population as well.

The reduction in new infections we find is based on expansion of MAT, NSP, HCT, and scale-up of ART among PWID. This involved reaching 20 percent coverage with each intervention, which is ambitious given current criminalization of drug use in Kenya and a base of currently low coverage levels of MAT, NSP, and HCT among PWID.

Criminalization of injecting drug use has led to marginalization of this population, preventing access to care and prevention services for PWID, and preventing health practitioners from providing supportive programs for PWID. Marginalization further increases risk of poor health outcomes for PWID. Based on the historical barriers to access and provision of services for PWID, it is reasonable to believe that none of the intervention scale-up or impacts modeled here can be realized if punitive policies against PWID persist. Such developments must be intensified and change implemented.

Treatment for HIV is a powerful tool for prevention, alongside equal access to care programs; high numbers of infections may be averted among PWID, other MARPs, and those who network with these populations. Benefits, however, cannot be observed with discriminating access to ART. In the context of the HIV epidemic in Kenya, expansion of programs for PWID is both a human rights and public health imperative.

CHAPTER 7

Policy Perspectives

Discussion of Modeling Results Across the Case Studies

The four case studies described above represent geographic, epidemic, social, and political diversity. A mixed/generalized epidemic in sub-Saharan Africa is represented by Kenya; the established HIV epidemic among PWID in Eastern Europe is represented by Ukraine; the developing epidemic and a changing landscape of prevention programs in South Asia is represented by Pakistan; and a mature epidemic in Southeast Asia is represented by Thailand. In all areas, the prevalence of HIV among PWID is over 10 percent although the prevalence in the adult population varies from low to generalized levels.

Many countries have plans to scale-up ART in coming years. In this context, discovering HIV-positive PWID, keeping them in care, and transferring them to HIV treatment when eligible, in numbers proportionate to their share in the overall population of HIV-positive individuals is a challenge worth taking up. In all four of the countries we find that current coverage of HIV treatment and care among PWID is very low, broadly reflective of the situation in low and middle income countries. We find that scale-up of ART with equi-proportionate access to PWID over 2012–2015 can account for significant reductions in HIV infections in the adult population compared to a status quo with flat ART coverage.

The joint technical guide developed by various partners envisages a combination of nine interventions related to harm reductions that can help achieve maximum impact; we have considered four. Over the period from 2012–2015, impressive reductions in the number of new HIV infections were observed among PWID when highly effective PWID and ART programs were expanded to ambitious yet achievable targets, in comparison to a status quo for these four interventions. Specifically, we observed in Ukraine a 34 percent reduction; in Pakistan, 33 percent; Thailand, 35 percent; and Kenya, 56 percent.

We investigated a policy decision many countries face: should they consider the combination package of four interventions or just continue with ART scale-up in which PWID can gain a proportional share? In this context we again looked at the impact in terms of HIV incidence. With such combination expansion and high effectiveness, countries could avert significant number of HIV infections compared to ART alone over 2012 to 2015: Ukraine: 11,130, Pakistan: 6,330, Thailand: 1,570, and Kenya 1,300. Table 7.1 combines these observations with the incremental total cost issue, and summarizes the cost-effectiveness.

Table 7.1   Incremental Cost-Effectiveness Ratios (ICER) of Policies Spanning 2012–15, Expressed As US$ per Adult HIV Infection Averted

Case study	Scaling-up combination prevention (NSP, MAT, HCT, and ART[a]) compared to status quo[b]	Scaling-up combination prevention compared to just scaling-up ART[a,c]
Ukraine	$598–$5,105	$6,732–$9,221
Pakistan	$520–$8,299	$9,848–$15,300
Thailand	$404–$788	$5,403–$6,819
Kenya	$1,459–$1,600	$13,166–$19,412

Source: Authors.
Note: ART = antiretroviral therapy; HCT = HIV counseling and testing; MAT = medically assisted therapy; NSP = needle and syringe program.
a. ART scale-up with equi-proportionate access to PWID in the number of treatment slots.
b. Range based on two policies: first, scaling up ART and offering PWID an equi-proportionate share in treatment slots; second, a scale-up of all four key harm reduction interventions (including ART with equal share).
c. Range shown here is based on variation in the modeled effectiveness of individual policies, and as captured in the Goals model impact matrix.

Table 7.1 suggests that in a diverse group of LMIC, when policymakers consider increasing combination prevention involving four key harm reduction interventions—NSP, MAT, HCT for PWID, and ART—they can expect very cost-effective or at least cost-effective investments.

However, countries facing resource constraints may also consider stepwise scale-up, beginning with a single intervention or a subset of the interventions. For example, in the four case studies, we specifically analyzed scaling up ART first and providing access to PWID on an equi-proportionate basis, as a step in an overall scale-up path.

Box 7.1   Illustrative Comparison to Other Cost-Effectiveness Results from LMIC

From a study in Southern India, diverse estimates of cost per HIV infection averted were obtained:

        MSM program: ....US$232

        Trucker program: ....US$1,810

        Migrant Labor program: ....US$2,167

        Other programs: ....US$3,536–US$10,655

Source: Dandona, Kumar et al. 2010.
Note: MSM = men who have sex with men

Our case study analysis was limited to directly observable effects from the Goals model, i.e., new infections. In the case studies, we did not consider the benefit-cost proposition in scaling up these interventions, specifically related to averted costs of treatment and care for each person at risk prevented from becoming HIV infected. In Table 7.2, we address this lack by considering the counterfactual. What would be the costs of pre-ART and thereafter first and second-line ART in individuals who become HIV-infected in each country? We assumed an average of two years after discovery of seropositive status (given that most people are tested later in their disease course) in pre-ART care, and then an average of three years each in first- and second-line antiretroviral therapy. Costs of ART by line of therapy varied by country and declined each successive year, with Kenya and Pakistan costs lower than Ukraine and Thailand. For a single year cost of each line of treatment, we took the average annual cost across our estimates for the period 2011–2015. Cost of laboratory tests for all and opportunistic infection treatment for a proportion of patients were included (tuberculosis prophylaxis was included in Ukraine for most). Details are provided in Appendix A.

Table 7.2   Benefit-Cost Ratios of Policies Involving Highly Effective Harm Reduction, by Country

Case study	Scaling-up combination prevention (NSP, MAT, HCT, and ART[a]) compared to status quo	Scaling-up combination prevention compared to just scaling up ART[a]
Ukraine	0.72	0.54
Pakistan	0.33	0.28
Thailand	8.35	1.22
Kenya	1.72	0.21

Source: Authors.
Note: ART = antiretroviral therapy; HCT = HIV counseling and testing; MAT = medically assisted therapy; NSP = needle and syringe program.
a. ART scale-up with equi-proportionate access to PWID in the number of treatment slots.

Based on this counterfactual, we estimate the total averted cost for the cumulative number of averted HIV infections over 2012–2015, for the comparisons of policies in Table 7.2. Thailand has benefit-cost ratios in excess of one, and Ukraine and Kenya also have high ratios.

When interpreting the overall picture of how the PWID-specific interventions affect the risk of HIV in the adult population several details must be considered. The population prevalence of PWID and the adult prevalence of HIV are highly influential in this context. Among the case studies, Ukraine and Pakistan have the greatest populations of PWID and very high HIV prevalence rates among PWID. In these two countries, the highest quantum of averted infections among adults is observed.

While in countries such as Thailand and Kenya the PWID population is relatively smaller, the impact is smaller but still relatively cost-effective compared to current low rates of coverage. Where there is already a high prevalence of HIV among the general adult population, such as in Kenya, lower impacts and greater cost per infection averted among the adult population are likely to be observed. Counter to this, countries such as Ukraine and Thailand where the HIV prevalence among adults is low (less than one percent) compared to high prevalence among PWID, we see greater benefits in terms of infections averted among both PWID and the adult populations. Costs per infections averted in these countries are likely lower as established ART and PWID programs cost less to expand as systems are already in place. In Kenya and Pakistan, programs are starting from a very low base and must include start-up costs.

This highlights limitation to modeling analyses that are dependent on inputs. If we get inputs such as population size estimates correct, then we can get believable results; yet the variety of sampling and population size estimation techniques can produce drastically different estimates.

Costs of the basket of PWID interventions is also influenced by the population that is opioid-dependent, and thus by the population in need of MAT. This is exemplified by Thailand, where only about 30 percent of the PWID population is assumed to be opioid dependent and thus the number of people to be covered by this more expensive program is lower in comparison to other countries such as Kenya, where the majority of PWID inject opiates.

The most striking result of our analysis is the similarity observed across these heterogeneous epidemics in terms of the impact on the PWID population when ART and PWID-specific interventions were expanded together. Cumulative reductions over 30 percent in adult infections compared to status quo were observed in all four case studies highlighting the benefits and importance of targeted HIV prevention programs for PWID.

This high level of reduction is for the high-effectiveness scenario of expansion. It is unlikely that such effectiveness will be achieved as long as PWID are marginalized, burdened by stigma, and suffer punitive sanctions. Drug use is criminalized in some form in all four countries.

The Need to Scale Up: Policy and Human Rights Perspectives

The results of this study demonstrate some key realities for the future of the global response to HIV. U.S. Secretary of State Hillary Clinton, in a landmark 2011 speech at the U.S. National Institutes of Health, called for "an AIDS-Free Generation." The findings presented here make clear that an AIDS-free generation will not be possible unless HIV prevention, treatment, and care are taken to scale for PWID. Scale up of HIV prevention, treatment, and care services for PWID, however, faces numerous and multi-faceted barriers spanning a range of political, social, and health sector echelons. (Further details on these barriers for each key intervention may be found in Appendix B). Indeed, while much of the world is seeing declines in new HIV infections, the PWID-driven epidemics of Eastern Europe, Central Asia, and parts of South Asia; are among the few areas globally where HIV epidemics continue to expand in 2012 (UNAIDS 2010).

This difficult truth is most clearly evidenced by the situation of Pakistan, where interruptions of basic services for PWID over 2009–2011, including needle and syringe exchange programs, almost certainly contributed to the sharp rise in HIV prevalence among PWID in Pakistani cities with large numbers of injectors. To truly begin to control the global spread of HIV, expansion, not contraction, of these services will be required. In this light, the December 2011 re-instatement of the U.S. federal ban on funding for needle and syringe exchanges is a substantial setback for scale-up efforts in the global response.

An additional and substantive concern for efforts to address HIV among PWID has been the cancellation of Round 11 funding of the Global Fund to Fight AIDS, TB, and Malaria (GFATM). The GFATM has been a critical donor for countries with concentrated epidemics, particularly in Asia and the Former Soviet Union. The GFATM has been willing to support NSEP, medication assisted therapy, and ARV treatment for PWID. Grants have supported community efforts, through non-country coordination mechanism (non-CCMS) in harm reduction activities when governments were unwilling to support these activities, as was the case in Thailand when the Thai Drug

Users Network received GFATM support. Interruptions of GFATM support thus are likely to have a disproportionate impact on countries with significant HIV burdens among PWID, and must be urgently addressed if we are not to see resurgent spread of HIV among these populations, and declines in urgently needed services.

The urgency for scaling up well-targeted combined prevention and treatment efforts for PWID is all the more compelling as the results of this study demonstrate that such efforts are not only effective, but cost-effective. While we did not conduct specific fiscal space analysis, we believe that the scale-up of well-targeted PWID interventions should occur within the existing context of allocations to the HIV/AIDS response in LMIC and given the totality of priorities for prevention, treatment, and care. It may be useful to conduct further analysis to understand the total fiscal space and contextualize the amount of scale-up to the available resources.

Responding to HIV among PWID is highly desirable from both public health and human rights perspectives. From a public health perspective, investing resources in key high-risk groups accords with the most basic principles of the field—high burden populations must receive efforts commensurate with disease prevalence and incidence for public health efforts to succeed. Ignoring significant populations at risk is approach which will undermine any public health effort.

From a human rights perspective the imperatives are equally compelling. People who inject drugs are no less deserving of services than any other group. Indeed Paul Hunt, the U.N. Special Rapporteur on the Right to Health has asserted that harm reduction is a legal obligation of states which have committed to the right to health for citizens. Human rights principles underscore that persons with drug dependence or addiction do not lose any fundamental rights, including the right to health care services, by virtue of the dependency. This is true for PWID in detention and prison as well, for whom drug treatment and ARV services are a compelling human rights priority and an obligation of states, given the overall context of the HIV/AIDS response.

The scientific evidence presented here, the public health rationale, and the human rights imperatives are all in accord: we can and must do better for PWID, especially in countries where current investments are disproportionate to the burden of HIV/AIDS among this group and given the importance in prevention. The available tools are evidence-based, right affirming, and cost effective. What is required now is political will and a global consensus that this critical component of global HIV can no longer be ignored and under-re-sourced. All those who seek an 'AIDS-free generation' will need to engage in the effort to expand HIV prevention, treatment and care for people who inject drugs.

References

AHRN (2009). "Harm Reduction Scale-up in Thailand." *AHRNews* 46/47: 14–15.

Alistar, S. S., D. K. Owens, et al. (2011). "Effectiveness and Cost Effectiveness of Expanding Harm Reduction and Antiretroviral Therapy in a Mixed HIV Epidemic: A Modeling Analysis for Ukraine." *PLoS Med* 8 (3): e1000423.

Armstrong, G., M. Kermode, et al. (2010). "Opioid substitution therapy in Manipur and Nagaland, north-east India: Operational research in action." *Harm Reduction Journal* 7 (1): 29.

Audoin, B. and C. Beyrer (2012). "Russia's retrograde stand on drug abuse." *New York Times.* New York.

Azim, T., N. Hussein, et al. (2005). "Effectiveness of harm reduction programmes for injecting drug users in Dhaka city." *Harm Reduction Journal* 2(1): 22.

Baral, S., G. Trapence, et al. (2009). "HIV prevalence, risks for HIV infection, and human rights among men who have sex with men (MSM) in Malawi, Namibia, and Botswana." *PLoS One* 4(3): e4997.

Beletsky, L., L. E. Grau, et al. (2011a). "Prevalence, characteristics, and predictors of police training initiatives by US SEPs: building an evidence base for structural interventions." *Drug and Alcohol Dependence* 119 (1–2): 145–149.

Beletsky, L., L. E. Grau, et al. (2011b). "The roles of law, client race and program visibility in shaping police interference with the operation of US syringe exchange programs." *Addiction* 106 (2): 357–365.

Beletsky, L., G. Martinez, et al. (2012). "Mexico's northern border conflict: collateral damage to health and human rights of vulnerable groups." *Pan American Journal of Public Health.*

Bergenstrom, A. M. and A. S. Abdul-Quader (2010). "Injection drug use, HIV and the current response in selected low-income and middle-income countries." *AIDS* 24: S20.

Beyrer, C. (2000). War in the Blood: Sex, Politics, and AIDS in Southeast Asia, London, Bangkok, Zed Books, White Lotus, St. Martin's Press.

Beyrer, C. (2011a). "Safe injection facilities save lives." *The Lancet* 377 (9775): 1385–1386.

Beyrer, C., S. D. Baral, et al. (2010). "The expanding epidemics of HIV type 1 among men who have sex with men in low- and middle-income countries: diversity and consistency." *Epidemiol Rev* 32 (1): 137–151.

Beyrer, C., J. Jittiwutikarn, et al. (2003). "Drug use, increasing incarceration rates, and prison-associated HIV risks in Thailand." *AIDS and Behavior* 7 (2): 153–161.

Beyrer, C., K. Malinowska-Sempruch, et al. (2010a). "Time to act: a call for comprehensive responses to HIV in people who use drugs." *The Lancet* 376 (9740): 551–563.

Beyrer, C., K. Malinowska-Sempruch, et al. (2010b). "Time to act: a call for comprehensive responses to HIV in people who use drugs (Panel 1: Portugal - humanitarianism and pragmatism)." *The Lancet* 376 (9740): 551–563.

Beyrer, C., A. L. Wirtz, et al. (2011). *The Global HIV Epidemics among Men Who Have Sex with Men*, Washington, DC: World Bank.

Beyrer, C., Wirtz, A., Walker, D., Johns, B., Sifakis, F., Baral, S. (2011b). The Global HIV Epidemics among Men Who Have Sex with Men: Epidemiology, Prevention, Access to Care and Human Rights, Washington, DC: World Bank.

Bobrova, N., T. Rhodes, et al. (2006). "Barriers to accessing drug treatment in Russia: a qualitative study among injecting drug users in two cities." *Drug and Alcohol Dependence* 82 Suppl 1: S57–63.

Booth, R. E., W. E. K. Lehman, et al. (2009). "Interventions with injection drug users in Ukraine." *Addiction* 104 (11): 1864–1873.

Brooner, R., M. Kidorf, et al. (1998). "Drug abuse treatment success among needle exchange participants." *Public Health Reports* 113 Suppl 1: 129–139.

Burnett Institute (2010). *Harm Reduction in Asia*: "Progress Torwards Universal Access to Harm Reduction Services Among People Who Inject Drugs." Commissioned on behalf of The United Nations Regional Task Force on Injecting Drug Use and HIV/AIDS in Asia and the Pacific.

CCM Pakistan (2009). "The Global Fund to fight AIDS,Tuberculosis, and Malaria: Proposal Form" - Round 9. Islamabad.

Chawarski, M. C., M. Mazlan, et al. (2008). "Behavioral drug and HIV risk reduction counseling (BDRC) with abstinence-contingent take-home buprenorphine: a pilot randomized clinical trial." *Drug and Alcohol Dependence* 94 (1–3): 281–284.

Cheluget, B., G. Baltazar, et al. (2006). "Evidence for population level declines in adult HIV prevalence in Kenya." *Sexually Transmitted Infections* 82 Suppl 1: i21–26.

Coalition ARV4IDUs (2004). "Availability of ARV for injecting drug users: key facts." XV International AIDS Conference. Coalition ARV4IDUs satellite meeting: *HIV treatment for drug users-a realistic goal*, Bangkok: International AIDS Society.

Cook, C. (2010). Global State of Harm Reduction (2010). *Key Issues for Broadening the Response*. International Harm Reduction Association. London.

Dandona, L., S. P. Kumar, et al. (2010). "Cost-effectiveness of HIV prevention interventions in Andhra Pradesh state of India." *BMC Health Services Research* 10 (1): 117.

Dar, N. (2012). "Second generation surveillance in Pakistan - Antenatal HIV sero-surveillance study." *National AIDS Control Program*, Ministry of Health. Islamabad

Degenhardt, L., B. Mathers, et al. (2010). "Prevention of HIV infection for people who inject drugs: why individual, structural, and combination approaches are needed." *The Lancet* 376 (9737): 285–301.

Denison, J. A., K. R. O'Reilly, et al. (2008). "HIV voluntary counseling and testing and behavioral risk reduction in developing countries: a meta-analysis, 1990–2005." *AIDS and Behavior* 12 (3): 363–373.

EMCDDA (2010). "The State of the Drugs Problem in Europe." European Monitoring Centre for Drugs and Drug Addiction (EMCDDA). Luxembourg.

Emmanuel, F. (2012). State of HIV in Pakistan - *Results of SGS* - Round IV (Presentation). National AIDS Control Program, Ministry of Health. Islamabad.

Emmanuel, F. and T. Reza (2012). *Second Generation Surveillance in Pakistan - Preliminary Results, Round 4* (Presentation). Islamabad, National AIDS Control Program, Ministry of Health.

Fisher, D. G., A. M. Fenaughty, et al. (2003). "Needle exchange and injection drug use frequency: a randomized clinical trial." *Journal of Acquired Immune Deficiency Syndromes* 33 (2): 199–205.

Friedmann, P. D., T. A. D'Aunno, et al. (2000). "Medical and psychosocial services in drug abuse treatment: do stronger linkages promote client utilization?" *Health Services Research* 35 (2): 443–465.

Futures Institute (2011). HIV Unit Costs Database: http://032c73d.netsolhost.com/index.aspx.

Futures Institute. (2012). Spectrum - Policy Projection Modeling Tool. Version 4.47 Beta 19..

Geibel et al. (2011). Nairobi MARPs Report (unpublished). *Population Council*, Nairobi Kenya.

Geibel, S. (2011). "Drug Use and HIV in Kenya." *Regional Workshop on Drug Use and HIV in Africa*, June 13, 2011. Nairobi, Kenya.

GFATM (2011). "Implementation Letter, Program Grant Agreement Number: PKS-911-G14-H." Geneva, The Global Fund to Fight AIDS, Tuberculosis, and Malaria.

Gibson, D. R., N. M. Flynn, et al. (2001). "Effectiveness of syringe exchange programs in reducing HIV risk behavior and HIV seroconversion among injecting drug users." *AIDS* 15 (11): 1329.

Gouws, E., P. J. White, et al. (2006a). "Short term estimates of adult HIV incidence by mode of transmission: Kenya and Thailand as examples." *Sexually Transmitted.Infections.* 82 (suppl 3): iii51–iii55.

Gouws, E., P. J. White, et al. (2006b). "Short term estimates of adult HIV incidence by mode of transmission: Kenya and Thailand as examples." *Sexually Transmitted Infections* 82 (suppl 3): iii51–iii55.

Gowing, L., M. Farrell, et al. (2008). "Substitution treatment of injecting opioid users for prevention of HIV infection." *Cochrane Database of System Reviews 2.*

Hammett, T. M., N. Bartlett, et al. (2005). "Law enforcement influences on HIV prevention for injection drug users: Observation from a cross border project in China and Vietnam." *International Journal of Drug Policy* 16: 235–245.

HIV/AIDS, U. C. f. (2011). September 2011 *Update Datasheet on Substitution Maintenance Therapy in Regions.*

Human Rights Watch (2004). *Lessons not learned: Human rights abuses and HIV/AIDS in the Russian Federation.* Moscow.

Human Rights Watch (2006). "Rhetoric and risk: Human rights abuses impeding Ukraine's fight against HIV/AIDS". New York.

Hurley, R. (2010). "How Ukraine is tackling Europe's worst HIV epidemic." *BMJ* 341.

IDU Reference Group (2010). "Consensus Statement of the Reference Group to the United Nations on HIV and Injecting Drug Use." Secretariat of the Reference Group to the United Nations on HIV and Injecting Drug Use.

Institute of Medicine (2007). "Preventing HIV Infection Among Injecting Drug Users in High-Risk Countries: An Assessment of Evidence." Institute of Medicine, Washington, DC.

International Harm Reduction Association (2010). The Global State of Harm Reduction 2010: Key Issues for Broadening the Response. London, UK: IHRA.

IOM (2007). Preventing HIV Infection among Injecting Drug Users in High Risk Countries: An Assessment of the Evidence. Washington, D.C.: *Institute of Medicine of The National Academies Press* (IOM), Committee on the Prevention of HIV Infection among Injecting Drug Users in High-Risk Countries.

Judice, N. (2012). *Use of Naltrexone and its Formulations in the Treatment of Opioid Dependence in the Russian Federation: Situation Analysis*. Washington, DC: Futures Group, Health Policy Project.

Jurgens, R. and G. Betteridge (2005). "Prisoners who inject drugs: public health and human rights imperatives." *Health and Human Rights* 8 (2): 46–74.

Jurgens, R. and J. Csete (2012). "In the name of treatment: ending abuses in compulsory drug detention centers." *Addiction* 107 (4): 689–691.

Jürgens, R., J. Csete, et al. (2010). "People who use drugs, HIV, and human rights." *The Lancet.*

Jurgens, R., M. Nowak, et al. (2011). "HIV and incarceration: prisons and detention." *Journal of the International AIDS Society* 14: 26.

Käll, K., U. Hermansson, et al. (2007). "The effectiveness of needle exchange programmes for HIV prevention—a critical review." *The Journal of Global Drug Policy and Practice* 1 (3).

Kawewa, J. (2005). Situational Analysis on HIV/AIDS in Kenya. *UNESCO.* Nairobi: University of Nairobi.

Kawichai, S., D. D. Celentano, et al. (2006). "HIV Voluntary Counseling and Testing and HIV Incidence in Male Injecting Drug Users in Northern Thailand: Evidence of an Urgent Need for HIV Prevention." *JAIDS Journal of Acquired Immune Deficiency Syndromes* 41 (2): 186–193 110.1097/1001.qai.0000179431.0000142284.0000179433e.

Kenya IDU TWG (2011). *Kenya IDU TWG Breakfast Meeting*, Nairobi (November 11, 2011).

Kerrigan, D., A. L. Wirtz, et al. (2012). *The Global Epidemics of HIV among Sex Workers*. T. Washington, DC: World Bank.

Khan, A. and A. Khan (2011). "Performance and coverage of HIV interventions for injection drug users: Insights from triangulation of programme, field and surveillance data from Pakistan." *The International Journal on Drug Policy.*

Khan, A. A. and A. Khan (2010). "The HIV Epidemic in Pakistan." *J Pak Medical Association* 60 (4): 300–307.

Kidorf, M. and V. L. King (2008). "Expanding the public health benefits of syringe exchange programs." *Canadian Journal of Psychiatry / Revue canadienne de psychiatrie* 53 (8): 487–495.

Kimani, J., R. Kaul, et al. (2008). "Reduced rates of HIV acquisition during unprotected sex by Kenyan female sex workers predating population declines in HIV prevalence." *AIDS* 22 (1): 131–137.

Kwon, J. A., J. Iversen, et al. (2009). "The impact of needle and syringe programs on HIV and HCV transmissions in injecting drug users in Australia: a model-based analysis." *JAIDS Journal of Acquired Immune Deficiency Syndromes* 51 (4): 462.

Lawrinson, P., R. Ali, et al. (2008). "Key findings from the WHO collaborative study on substitution therapy for opioid dependence and HIV/AIDS." *Addiction* 103 (9): 1484–1492.

Lei, Z., Y. Lorraine, et al. (2011). "Needle and syringe programs in Yunnan, China yield health and financial return." *BMC Public Health* 11.

MacArthur, G. J., Minozzi, S, Martin, N., Vickerman, P., Deren, S., and J. Bruneau, et al. Opiate substitution treatment and HIV transmission in people who inject drugs: systematic review and meta-analysis. BMJ 2012;345:e5945

Mahapatra, B., P. Goswami, et al. (2010). "Determinants of HIV prevalence among intravenous drug users (IDUs) in North-Eastern India: evidence from two rounds of surveys (Abstract no. THPE0381)." International AIDS Conference, Rome, *International AIDS Society.*

Martin, M., S. Vanichseni, et al. (2011). *Enrollment characteristics, follow-up, risk behavior, and assessing adherence of injecting drug users in a pre-exposure prophylaxis trial in Bangkok.* CROI 2011.

Mathers, B., L. Degenhardt, et al. (2008). "Global epidemiology of injecting drug use and HIV among people who inject drugs: a systematic review." *The Lancet* 372: 1733–1745.

Mathers, B. M., L. Degenhardt, et al. (2010). "HIV prevention, treatment, and care services for people who inject drugs: a systematic review of global, regional, and national coverage." *The Lancet* 375 (9719): 1014–1028.

Mattick, R. P., C. Breen, et al. (2009). "Methadone maintenance therapy versus no opioid replacement therapy for opioid dependence." *Cochrane Database of Systematic Reviews* (3): CD002209.

Mattick, R. P., J. Kimber, et al. (2008). "Buprenorphine maintenance versus placebo or methadone maintenance for opioid dependence." *Cochrane Database of Systematic Reviews* (2): CD002207.

Milloy, M. J., N. Fairbairn, et al. (2010). "Overdose experiences among injection drug users in Bangkok, Thailand." *Harm Reduction J* 7: 9.

Ministry of Health Ukraine (2010). *Ukraine: National Report on Monitoring Progress Towards the UNGASS Declaration of Commitment on HIV/AIDS.* Kyiv.

Ministry of Public Health Thailand (2010). *Country Progress Report.* Bangkok, UNGASS.

NACC and NASCOP (2011). National HIV Indicators for Kenya: 2010. Nairobi, Kenya, *National AIDS Coordination Council & the National AIDS/STD Control Programme.*

NACC and World Bank (2009). Kenya HIV Prevention Response and Modes of Transmission Analysis. Nairobi, Kenya, *National AIDS Control Council.*

NACP (2005). HIV Second Generation Surveillance in Pakistan - National Report Round 1. Islamabad, *National AIDS Control Program,* Ministry of Health.

NACP (2007). HIV Second Generation Surveillance in Pakistan - National Report Round 2 (2006–2007). Islamabad, *National AIDS Control Program, Ministry of Health.*

NACP (2008). HIV Second Generation Surveillance in Pakistan - National Report Round 3. Islamabad, *National AIDS Control Program, Ministry of Health.*

NACP (2010a). HIV Second Generation Surveillance in Pakistan - National Report on Young Individuals from High Risk Groups. Islamabad, *National AIDS Control Program, Ministry of Health.*

NACP (2010b). UNGASS Pakistan Report: Progress Report on the Declaration of Commitment on HIV/AIDS for the United Nations General Assembly Special Session on HIV/AIDS. Islamabad, *National AIDS Control Program, Ministry of Health.*

Nai Zindagi (2008). *The Hidden Truth.* Islamabad, Pakistan.

NASCOP (2009). *Kenya National AIDS Strategic Plan 2010–2013 - Delivering on Universal Access to Services.* Nairobi: Office of the President.

Ndetei, D. (2004). *Study on the assessment of the linkages between drug abuse, injecting drug abuse and HIV/AIDS in Kenya: a rapid situation assessment.* Nairobi: UNODC.

Needle, R. and L. Zhao (2010). *HIV prevention among injection drug users: Strengthening US support for core interventions.* C. G. H. P. Center. Washington, DC.

Odek-Ogunde, M. (2004). *World Health Organization phase II drug injecting study: behavioural and seroprevalence (HIV, HBV, HCV) survey among injecting drug users in Nairobi.* Nairobi, Kenya: World Health Organization.

Pakistan Harm Reduction Technical Advisory Committee (2012). *HIV among People who Inject Drugs in Pakistan: Rising Prevalence and Urgency of a Scaled-up Response in 2012.* Islamabad.

Pang, L., Y. Hao, et al. (2007). "Effectiveness of first eight methadone maintenance treatment clinics in China." *AIDS* 21 Suppl 8: S103–107.

PEPFAR (2010). *Comprehensive HIV Prevention for People Who Inject Drugs*, Revised Guidance. Washington, DC.

Perngmark, P., S. Vanichseni, et al. (2008). "The Thai HIV/AIDS epidemic at 15 years: sustained needle sharing among southern Thai drug injectors." *Drug Alcohol Dependance* 92 (1–3): 183–190.

Pollini, R. A., R. Lozada, et al. (2010). "Barriers to pharmacy-based syringe purchase among injection drug users in Tijuana, Mexico: a mixed methods study." *AIDS and Behavior* 14 (3): 679–687.

Qian, H. Z., C. Hao, et al. (2008). "Impact of methadone on drug use and risky sex in China." *Journal of Substance Abuse Treatment* 34 (4): 391–397.

Quan, V. M., T. Vongchak, et al. (2007). "Predictors of mortality among injecting and non-injecting HIV-negative drug users in northern Thailand." *Addiction* 102 (3): 441–446.

Rhodes, T. and D. Hedrich, Eds. (2010). *Harm Reduction: Evidence, Impacts and Challenges.* Luxembourg: European Monitoring Centre for Drugs and Drug Addiction.

Rhodes, T., L. Platt, et al. (2006). "Street policing, injecting drug use and harm reduction in a Russian city: a qualitative study of police perspectives." *Journal of Urban Health: Bulletin of the New York Academy of Medicine* 83 (5): 911–925.

Rouanvong, W. (2007). "*Opening Speech.*" 9th ICPA Conference, Bangkok.

Schaub, M., V. Chtenguelov, et al. (2010). "Feasibility of buprenorphine and methadone maintenance programmes among users of home made opioids in Ukraine." *The International al Journal on Drug Policy* 21 (3): 229–233.

Schwartländer, B., J. Stover, et al. (2011). "Towards an improved investment approach for an effective response to HIV/AIDS." *The Lancet* 377: 2031–2041.

Sharma, M., E. Oppenheimer, et al. (2009). "A situation update on HIV epidemics among people who inject drugs and national responses in South-East Asia Region." *AIDS* 23 (11): 1405–1413.

Shulga, L. (2011). "Sexual HIV transmission among PWID." *Regional Workshop on Drug Use and HIV in Eastern Europe and Central Asia*, Kiev.

Singh, K., P. Brodish, et al. (2011). "A Venue-Based Approach to Reaching MSM, IDUs and the General Population with VCT: A Three Study Site in Kenya." *AIDS and Behavior.*

Strathdee, S. A., T. B. Hallett, et al. (2010). "HIV and risk environment for injecting drug users: the past, present, and future." *The Lancet.*

Strathdee, S. A., E. P. Ricketts, et al. (2006). "Facilitating entry into drug treatment among injection drug users referred from a needle exchange program: Results from a community-based behavioral intervention trial." *Drug and Alcohol Dependence* 83 (3): 225–232.

Sued, O., C. Schreiber, et al. (2011). "HIV drug and supply stock-outs in Latin America." *The Lancet Infectious Diseases* 11(11): 810–811.

Thaisri, H., J. Lerwitworapong, et al. (2003). "HIV infection and risk factors among Bangkok prisoners, Thailand: a prospective cohort study." *BMC Infectious Diseases* 3 (1): 25.

The A2 Thailand and the Thai Working Group on HIV/AIDS Projections (2008). *The Asian Epidemic Model (AEM) Projections for HIV/AIDS in Thailand: 2005–2025.* Bangkok, Family Health International,Bureau of AIDS, TB and STI, Department of Disease Control, MOPH.

Tun, W., J. Okal, et al. (2011). "HIV Prevalence and Injection Behaviors Among Injecting Drug Users in Nairobi: *Results from a 2011 Bio-Behavioral Study Using Respondent-Driven Sampling* (MOLBPE049)." 6th IAS Conference on HIV Pathogenesis and Treatment and Prevention, Rome.

Uhlmann, S., M. J. Milloy, et al. (2010). "Methadone maintenance therapy promotes initiation of antiretroviral therapy among injection drug users." *Addiction* 105n(5): 907–913.

UNAIDS (2005). *Update on the Global HIV/AIDS Pandemic*. Geneva.

UNAIDS (2008). *2008 Report on the global AIDS epidemic*. Geneva.

UNAIDS (2010). *Report on the Global AIDS Epidemic*. Geneva.

UNODC (2007). *HIV and Prisons in Sub-Saharan Africa: Opportunities for Action*. Geneva.

UNODC (2009). *From coercion to cohesion: Treating drug dependence through health care, not punishment* (Discussion paper), Vienna. United Nations Office on Drugs and Crime.

UNODC (2012). Respondent Driven Sampling (RDS) Study and Population Size Estimation in Nairobi and Kenyan Coast Province in 2011. *Rapid Situation Assessment on HIV among IDUs in Kenya*. Nairobi, United Nations.

USAID (2010). *Thailand: Overview of the HIV Epidemic and the National HIV/AIDS surveillance*. Bangkok.

USAID, WHO, et al. (2007). *Module 6: Managing ART in Injecting Drug Users* - Participant Manual. Jakarta.

VAHC, UNAIDS, et al. (2010). *Evaluation of the Epidemiological Impact of Harm Reduction Programs on HIV in Vietnam.*, Vietnam Administration for HIV/AIDS Control, UNAIDS, World Bank, University of New South Wales, and Partnership for Epidemic Analysis.

Vitek, C. (2011). "HIV and IDU in Ukraine." *Regional Workshop on Drug Use and HIV in Eastern Europe and Central Asia*, Kiev.

Werb, D., E. Wood, et al. (2008). "Effects of police confiscation of illicit drugs and syringes among injection drug users in Vancouver." *The International Journal on Drug Policy* 19 (4): 332–338.

Weller S, Davis-Beaty K. Condom effectiveness in reducing heterosexual HIV transmission (Art. No.: CD003255). *Cochrane Database of Systematic Reviews 2002*.

WHO (2012). *Cost-effectiveness thresholds*. Geneva.

WHO and UNODC (2009). *Guidance on Testing and Counselling for HIV in Settings Attended by People who Inject Drugs: Improving Access to Treatment, Care, and Prevention*, World Health Organization and United Nations Office on Drugs and Crime.

WHO, UNODC, et al. (2009). *Technical Guide for Countries to Set Targets for Universal Access to HIV Prevention, Treatment and Care for Injecting Drug Users*. Geneva, World Health Organization, UNODC, UNAIDS.

Wiessing, L., G. Likatavicius, et al. (2009). "Associations between availability and coverage of HIV-prevention measures and subsequent incidence of diagnosed HIV infection among injection drug users." *American Journal of Public Health* 99 (6): 1049.

Wodak, A. and A. Cooney (2004). *Effectiveness of sterile needle and syringe programming in reducing HIV/AIDS among injecting drug users*. Geneva.

Wolfe, D. (2007). "Paradoxes in antiretroviral treatment for injecting drug users: access, adherence and structural barriers in Asia and the former Soviet Union." *The International Journal on Drug Policy* 18 (4): 246–254.

Wolfe, D., M. P. Carrieri, et al. "Treatment and care for injecting drug users with HIV infection: a review of barriers and ways forward." *The Lancet* 376 (9738): 355–366.

Wolfe, D., M. P. Carrieri, et al. (2010). "Treatment and care for injecting drug users with HIV infection: a review of barriers and ways forward." *The Lancet* 376 (9738): 355–366.

Wood, E., R. S. Hogg, et al. (2008). "Highly active antiretroviral therapy and survival in HIV-infected injection drug users." *JAMA: The Journal of the American Medical Association* 300 (5): 550–554.

World Bank (2010). *World Development Indicators.* Washington, D.C: World Bank.

APPENDIX A

Unit Costs of Interventions

Unit Costs for PWID-specific Interventions

In the case of Ukraine and Thailand, it was assumed that NSP and HCT for PWID had achieved substantial economies of scale and had settled into a steady-state level of design where variation in costs per PWID reached would not be significant as scale of coverage increased. This was not the case in Kenya and Pakistan, where programs are beginning and there is some start-up and capacity-building cost. Data for unit costs of HCT and NSP in Pakistan came from documents related to the GFATM Round 10 grant. For others, we used values from a recent multi-country study (Schwartländer, Stover et al. 2011)

Table A.1	Unit costs, Ukraine (2011 US$)			
	2012	2013	2014	2015
PWID: HCT	16	16	16	16
PWID: NSP	10	10	10	10
PWID MAT[a]	907	874	840	806

Source: Schwartländer, Stover et al. 2011
Note: HCT = HIV counseling and testing; MAT = medically assisted therapy; NSP = needle and syringe program.
a. Declining cost schedule with increasing coverage.

Table A.2   Unit Costs, Kenya (2011 US$)

	2012	2013	2014	2015
PWID: HCT	14	14	13	12
PWID: NSP	29	27	26	24
PWID MAT[a]	959	908	858	807

Source: Schwartländer, Stover et al. 2011
Note: HCT = HIV counseling and testing; MAT = medically assisted therapy; NSP = needle and syringe program.
a. Declining cost schedule with increasing coverage.

Table A.3   Unit Costs, Pakistan (2011 US$)

	2012	2013	2014	2015
PWID: HCT	15	15	15	15
PWID: NSP	67	39	39	39
PWID MAT[a]	907	874	840	806

Source: Schwartländer, Stover et al. 2011.
Note: HCT = HIV counseling and testing; MAT = medically assisted therapy; NSP = needle and syringe program.
a. Declining cost schedule with increasing coverage.

Table A.4   Unit Costs, Thailand (2011 US$)

	2012	2013	2014	2015
PWID: HCT	94	90	87	84
PWID: NSP	100	98	96	94
PWID MAT	1,009	1,009	1,009	1,009

Source: Schwartländer, Stover et al. 2011.
Note: HCT = HIV counseling and testing; MAT = medically assisted therapy; NSP = needle and syringe program.

Table A.5   Costs of Support Functions Added on Total Costs Including ART (All Cases)

Policy and administration	5%
Research	1%
Monitoring and evaluation	1%
Human resources	2%

Source: Schwartländer, Stover et al. 2011.
Note: ART = antiretroviral therapy.

Unit Costs for Antiretroviral Treatment

Table A.6   Unit Costs, Kenya and Pakistan (2011 US$)

	2012	2013	2014	2015
First line ART drugs	133.5	132.3	131.2	130
Second line ART drugs	501.5	384.3	267.2	150
Lab costs	155	146.7	138.3	130
Drug and lab costs for opportunistic infections	160	160	160	160
Cotrimoxazole prophylaxis	4	4	4	4

Source: Authors; Global Fund Round 10 grant proposals.
Note: ART = antiretroviral therapy.

Table A.7   Unit Costs, Ukraine (2011 US$)

	2012	2013	2014	2015
First line ART drugs	140	138	137	135
Second line ART drugs	1151	924	696	469
Lab costs	169.7	159.3	148.9	138.5
Drug and lab costs for opportunistic infections	349	349	349	349
Cotrimoxazole prophylaxis	1	1	1	1

Source: Authors.
Note: ART = antiretroviral therapy.

Table A.8   Unit Costs, Thailand (2011 US$)

	2012	2013	2014	2015
First line ART drugs	162	157	152	148
Second line ART drugs	1479	1435	1392	1350
Lab costs	190	180	170	160
Drug and lab costs for opportunistic infections	558	558	558	558
Cotrimoxazole prophylaxis	4	4	4	4

Source: Authors.
Note: ART = antiretroviral therapy.

Other Parameters

Kenya/Pakistan	Probability of opportunistic infection per year: 0.2
Ukraine/Thailand	Probability of opportunistic infection per year: 0.1

Source: Authors.

APPENDIX B

Barriers and Constraints to Provision and Scale-up of Key Interventions for PWID

Intervention	Barriers: Costs and Resources	Political	Policing	Other Structural	Social	Health Sector
HIV Counseling and Testing	↑ Low cost, can be integrated into a range of programs and outreach to maximize coverage and cost efficiency	↑ Required reporting of the mode of HIV transmission in some setting	↑ Policing of outreach that includes HCT for PWID, may indirectly impact access to/uptake of HCT available through outreach	↑ Homelessness and/or lack of transportation reduces access to HCT centers and receipt of test results	↑ Dual stigmatization (experienced or perceived) of drug use and HIV infection (Human Rights Watch 2006; Beletsky, Martinez et al. 2012)	↑ Stigmatization of PWID in health sector (Beletsky, Martinez et al. 2012) ↑ Blood-based HIV testing challenging for long-term injectors ↑ Lack of confidentiality: staff may violate patient's privacy and disclose HIV status (Human Rights Watch 2006)
Antiretroviral Therapy	↔ High cost but covers large, general population ↑ Drug stock-outs in low resourced settings may inhibit provision or lead to treatment interruption of general and IDU populations in need of ART (Sued, Schreiber et al. 2011)	↓ Few political barriers	Little policing targeted to ART; however, incarceration of HIV+ PWID can lead to treatment interruptions where prisons are low resourced	↑ Homelessness, poverty, lack of transportation may reduce access to treatment and adherence	↑ Dual stigmatization (experienced or perceived) of drug use and HIV infection[a] (Human Rights Watch 2006; Mathers, Degenhardt et al. 2010)	↑ Some countries require urine specimen prior to providing ART ↑ Clinician concern that active drug users will not be adherent to treatment and may lead to resistance (Wolfe 2007) ↓ Provision of MAT (Wood, Hogg et al. 2008; Uhlmann, Milloy et al. 2010) or integration into NSP (Wolfe 2007) can lead to increased initiation and adherence to ART

(continued next page)

(continued)

Intervention	Barriers: Costs and Resources	Political	Policing	Other Structural	Social	Health Sector
Medically Assisted Therapy	↔ Moderate cost for coverage of smaller opioid using population but considered cost-effective for benefits(Needle and Zhao 2010)	↑ Politically controversial, often based on the assumption that methadone replaces one drug with another(Needle and Zhao 2010; Audoin and Beyrer 2012)[b] ↑ Specific legislation in some countries prohibits MAT (Needle and Zhao 2010; Audoin and Beyrer 2012)	↑ Incarceration of PWID can interrupt treatment and recovery of PWID, particularly where prison systems lack appropriate treatment programs for inmates(UNODC 2009) or risk relapse with exposure to drug use within the prison setting (Jurgens and Betteridge 2005; UNODC 2007; Cook 2010; Geibel 2011; Jurgens, Nowak et al. 2011)	↑ Homelessness, poverty/lack of insurance, lack of transportation may reduce access to MAT centers (Brooner, Kidorf et al. 1998; Friedmann, D'Aunno et al. 2000; Strathdee, Ricketts et al. 2006)	↑ Discrimination and stigma of PWID (perceived or experienced) may lead to avoidance of available MAT by PWID (Human Rights Watch 2004; Hammett, Bartlett et al. 2005; Human Rights Watch 2006; Wolfe 2007)	↑ MAT restricted to low dose and/or detoxification tapers in some settings* (Beyrer 2000) ↑ Compulsory treatment centers or other rehabilitation services may not be resourced to provide ART to residents(Needle and Zhao 2010) ↑ Restriction of providers who can prescribe MAT in some settings ↑ Name-based reporting required for registration in MAT may provoke PWID to avoid services (Needle and Zhao 2010)

(continued next page)

(continued)

Intervention	Barriers: Costs and Resources	Political	Policing	Other Structural	Social	Health Sector
	↓ Scale up of treatment may reduce other costs such as drug treatment, prison/detention costs (Wolfe, Carrieri et al.)	↑ Harm reduction organizations targeted for providing services or information, effectively prevents provision of MAT (Audoin and Beyrer 2012)				↑ Perceived efficacy of treatment (Bobrova, Rhodes et al. 2006) ↓ Treatment motivation and entry can be improved with integration into other outreach and NSPs (Strathdee, Ricketts et al. 2006; Kidorf and King 2008)
Medically Assisted Therapy		↑ Employment restrictions prevents uptake of MAT by PWID (Needle and Zhao 2010) ↓ Decriminalization of drug use may increase access to treatment[c]				

(continued next page)

(continued)

Intervention	Barriers: Costs and Resources	Political	Policing	Other Structural	Social	Health Sector
Needle and Syringe Programs	↓ Low cost for coverage of PWID population (Werb, Wood et al. 2008)	↑ Controversial in some settings (less so, compared to MAT), mostly associated with misconception that NSP leads to increased drug use[d]	↑ NSP sites easily targeted by police, may include harassment, violence, and/or arrest of PWID (Human Rights Watch 2006; Rhodes, Platt et al. 2006; Werb, Wood et al. 2008; Beletsky, Grau et al. 2011a; Beletsky, Grau et al. 2011b) ↑ Harassment of outreach workers or peer educators (Human Rights Watch 2006)	↑ Transportation to NSP sites ↓ *Mobile outreach methods of NSP may overcome distance and transportation challenges*	↑ Discrimination of PWID: PWID may avoid NSPs out of fear they will be identified as PWID Local community opposition to operation of NSPs in neighborhoods due to fear that it will encourage drug use or trafficking (Needle and Zhao 2010)	↑ Pharmacy laws may prohibit dispensing or possessing syringes without a valid prescription ↑ Discrimination within pharmacies or pharmacist fear of repercussion by authorities, even where syringe programs and over-the-counter programs are sanctioned prevent access to clean syringes by PWID (Pollini, Lozada et al. 2010) ↑ Health officials and staff do not view NSP as part of a continuum of care

Source: Authors.
Note: ART = antiretroviral therapy; HCT = HIV counseling and testing; MAT = medically assisted therapy; NSP = needle and syringe program.
a. Globally, only 4 of 100 PWID infected with HIV are receiving ART (Degenhardt, Mathers et al. 2010) "Low dose or tapering do not fall under best practices guidelines for MAT.
b. Cochrane reviews have reported the effectiveness of methadone and buprenorphine for reducing heroin use (Mattick, Kimber et al. 2008; Mattick, Breen et al. 2009).
c. Decriminalization of personal use in Portugal has demonstrated an increase from 32,000 to 38,5000 people in treatment between 2002–08 (Beyrer, Malinowska-Sempruch et al. 2010b).
d. Evidence from trials in the US (and other countries) have demonstrated there is no increase in drug use with NSP (Fisher, Fenaughty et al. 2003).

www.ingramcontent.com/pod-product-compliance
Lightning Source LLC
Chambersburg PA
CBHW071053280326
41928CB00050B/2459